MOPSI

*The All in One Tool to Clear the
Cobwebs out of Your Brain*

NANCY L SWAYZEE, MES, NMT
EDITED BY FRANK CARTON

ISBN: 1536984132
ISBN 13: 9781536984132
Library of Congress Control Number: 2016913091
CreateSpace Independent Publishing Platform
North Charleston, South Carolina

DEDICATION

*I dedicate this book to my granddaughter, Madelyn Kylee Bond,
without whom this book would not have been possible.
Her personal injury, her resilience, her willingness to work, and
her amazing spirit are what inspired me to write this book.*

■ ■ ■

ACKNOWLEDGEMENTS

First and foremost, I want to acknowledge and thank my fabulous editor, Frank Carton. His patience with my particular writing quirks is a testimony to his professionalism. A fellow writer and dear friend, he not only corrected my punctuation errors, he restructured my run on sentences. My excitement about this subject lends to my going on and on and on . . .

I must give special mention to a small business, No Problem, here in Grass Valley. It is a computer-help, repair, straighten-out-messes, teach-their-patrons, and clear-up-viruses business. Three great guys, Rob, Chris, and Mike, have really allowed this book to be possible by getting me out of more computer messes than you could imagine. My undying gratitude to them for their help.

FOREWORD

I thought this would be a good place to explain the "writing quirks" I referred to in the Acknowledgements. I tend to write like I talk … which is a lot. With all this talking, I need to take breaths, hence, the commas.

Because I must have been "Out to Lunch" during basic English Grammar in high school, somehow I never absorbed the basics of punctuation. Although my speaking grammar is close to flawless, I have to admit that I LOVE dots, dashes, italics, parentheses, ellipses, hyphens, quotations marks, semicolons, and colons! The combination of my excitement about the subject, together with the speed with which my brain jumps around, explain all the parenthetical information. I no more start to explain something, then I think of something else (hopefully connected) that I need to add.

Regardless, I'm hoping the interest value, as well as the good intentions that began this book, will allow you to overlook my flaws and see the information as flawless. If the over-punctuation [*sic*] tends to make you itchy or exasperated, put the book down, walk around the room, take deep breaths, and come back to it when you're ready. By the way, IMPORTANT! Make sure you get your physicians "okay" before you do any of the exercises. Take it with you and let them see what they are.

nls

TABLE OF CONTENTS

INTRODUCTION

Just for Starters . . .

It seems we have always been fascinated with what is inside our head. Hippocrates, Plato and Aristotle had different views on what exactly the contents inside the skull did. It wasn't until Galen, the Roman physician, put together, that injury to the head of a gladiator often resulted in loss of some kind of function within the body. It took until the late 1960s for the *Society for Neuroscience* to be established. The study of the connection between the nervous system and the brain began to expand.

Still, it is common in human practice to see things as separate, hence, the era of specialization. Studying the separate components of the functions of both the body and the brain, has allowed for in-depth research of individual components of disciplines such as neurology, psychiatry, neuropathology, and neurobiology. Neurobiology has probably come closest to studying the integration of the body and the brain. This book is about the *connection* and the *integration* of the functions of the *whole body* and the *whole brain*. It is a brain training book about *using* your body to facilitate better *use* of your brain. Whatever the reason you found this, it can have the power to change your life for the better.

Recognizing the potential we have to improve, increase, strengthen and sharpen our cognitive abilities, by understanding the crucial link between *using* our body and *using* our brain . . . the fact that they are inseparable opens a world of possibility you may not have known was there. This is a program that *uses* the whole body in a specific way that *uses* the whole brain. It's also a program that *benefits* the whole body by the specific nature of the use.

This is not a breathing program, but it does involve the breath. It is a program, through physical movement, that promotes the increase of oxygen in the blood that nourishes the whole body and the whole brain. The purpose of this book is to offer a unique science-based method that is designed to slow down the cognitive decline associated with aging. Although this program has not been clinically evaluated yet (except on myself), I see results every day, not only in myself, but in my students. The entire concept was and continues to be based on the latest neuroscience as it is released to the public. In addition, I search the web for any of the newest research in the pipeline.

MOPSI ???

So the first thing I should do, is tell you what MOPSI stands for. It an acronym for Movement - Oxygenation - Play - Stimulation - Interaction: MOPSI, the five things absolutely necessary for both physical and mental and emotional health. This fully-packed book has a variety of topics for the curious reader. I say curious because the science in this book is definitely directed toward the reader who loves to learn.

Not an exercise book, it is full of active movement and physical activities that allow a scenic tour through the interaction between the body and the brain *during* exercise. I explain some of those mysterious processes that the body and brain do to keep us functioning, without any direct commands or instructions from us. I wrote the book for a broad audience, particularly men and women in their 60s, but it is as important for someone in their 40s or 50s, who may be witnessing the slow cognitive decline of a parent or a spouse. At a workshop I recently gave to professionals primarily under 60 who were caring for elderly parents . . . they couldn't wait to get their hands on this book.

This program is perfect for someone who has just been diagnosed with Type II Diabetes, or any other disease that is positively impacted by the addition of regular exercise at a moderately low level. It is appropriate for anyone who has a large amount of weight on them, because it's slow and gentle and can be a great "fill-in" between harder workouts, and allows for a period of maintenance at whatever level they have achieved. People who are seriously overweight have probably not been moving much. That means they have not only been short-changing their brains of oxygen, they haven't been producing any of the BDNFs you will learn about in Chapter Three. I am offering some solutions.

The addition of the DVD of the exercises, demonstrated by myself and a couple of other older adults, is important. It not only gives enormous value and convenience to the reader, but it allows you to *see* how to *safely* and *effectively* do the exercises. Using your eyes and ears to initiate the processing of information is how we develop from infants into thinking, functioning adults!

The written exercises reach the brain in a way the visual ones can't -- and vice versa. Because you're using your language centers to read them, you are unconsciously building images in your mind. More good news: if you read them out-loud, you get twice the benefit. You are *actively* using your speech centers and your auditory cortex. When you see the exercises on the DVD, this either reinforces or corrects what that image is. Now you can go back to the written description, and it all makes sense!

First, I am the author -- a 77 year old -- full of energy, enthusiasm and passion for what I do. Most important of all, this is a program adaptable to any and every physical condition. It's perfect for seniors living in an assisted-living situation, even if a fitness program is being provided, it's often not enough to offset the ravages of time and the normal cognitive decline associated with aging. These are small exercises that can be done by someone confined to a wheelchair or who is unsteady on their feet and needs to exercise sitting down. They take very little space, so they can be done in small spaces like a small apartment or an office cubicle. Some of the exercises can even be done in bed! Here is a quote from a male patient with MS, whom I worked with for about two years. I went to his house twice a week and we worked in his small living room, with a grand piano, an organ and two large dog crates. I asked him to tell me how he felt about the exercises I was teaching him.

He said: "As more and more things were taken away from me (the ability to do), I just curled up into a little ball and became more and more isolated. After my fall on July 4th, two years ago - I never expected to even reach 65 years of age. What has changed is hope . . . light at the end of the tunnel. I discovered I could still have some of the things I loved (playing music), in my life. It was learning I could just learn to do them in a new way. Learning to do things differently."

The program can be interactive, like Chair Dancing and Ball Room Dancing, (things Bob and his girlfriend learned to do), because many of the exercises are the most fun when done with a partner. They are a great opportunity for play time between grandparents and their grandchildren, and very important, between spouses!

How did I make the shift from the Breathworks rehabilitative exercises to working with brain injury and neurological conditions? After injuring my back in early 1988 in Colorado, I created and developed the original CORE exercises that led to my own rehabilitation. Moving back to California after the birth of my granddaughter, I began the process of getting the certifications and credentials necessary, and began teaching the CORE Exercises through Tahoe Forest Hospital in Truckee, CA. In 1991 I opened a private practice as a rehabilitative exercise therapist, specializing in back injuries.

In 1993, son and my granddaughter, then four and one half years old, were involved in a tragic accident that resulted in life altering injuries to them both and a Traumatic Brain Injury for her. After their initial hospitalization and therapies, they returned to California and asked me if I would move to a cottage on their property and work with Madelyn. During the next eight years, while working with my granddaughter daily, I read everything I could get my hands on about the brain, exercise the specific modalities for TBI and stroke rehabilitation. Fortunately, all the ground breaking discoveries about the brain were taking place at the same time. In the intervening years, I worked with other patients with brain injuries, Parkinson's disease, Stroke, MS and cerebral palsy. All gained increased abilities and improved function, whether the ability to move or to breathe. Some improvements were large, some small, but all improved the quality of their lives.

I said this book was written for people who are curious and still interested in learning, because it is for those who are open to new approaches to old problems. Most importantly, those who want to keep or re-capture that young, vital energy and enthusiasm for life they once had. If you took a chance and bought this book, Thank You. If someone gave it to you, and you decided to open it, Thank You. However you came upon it, I hope it offers you something of interest and value, and most importantly, makes a difference in your life. It certainly has in mine.

Nancylister Swayzee

1

ALL SYSTEMS GO

When was the last time you thought about your brain? (Now, thinking about your brain is a little like the chicken and the egg thing, but I mean *really*, do you *think* about your brain?) As far as that goes, when was the last time you *thought* about your body? I don't mean body image or "Do I have a deadly disease?" I mean *think* about, wonder about, how amazing these two things are -- consider how difficult living would become if they weren't both operating at maximum capacity. The perfection of the human body/human brain connection is as fascinating as quantum physics! (In fact, it IS quantum physics!) In Michael Sweeny's brilliant book *Brain: THE COMPLETE MIND HOW IT DEVELOPS, HOW IT WORKS, AND HOW TO KEEP IT SHARP,* he compares it to quantum physics by the unpredictability of our thinking processes. It's been called the Chaos Theory. He says, "Precise measurement -- the basis for a physically deterministic world -- becomes impossible at the smallest scale, i.e., electrons and neutrons, etc. There is always uncertainty, and thus we can never fully know our world -- or the brain."

Sadly, we abuse them with too much food, drugs, and alcohol, bad mouthing them all the time with remarks like: "Boy, am I stupid." "I HATE my body." "How could I have been so dumb?" Here's a little secret . . . Your brain and body *hear* you. You're sending them the wrong message. They need to know you care about them. We allow them both to lie idle while we mindlessly punch keypads with our thumbs or fingers: trancelike, motionless, doodling on iPhones, iPads and iTunes.

The NBC Nightly News released the results of a Harvard study that showed that people who let their minds wander from their activities at the moment aren't happy. Their minds are often busy scanning their "To-Do Lists," running their "should haves, could haves," through their minds. The experts' conclusion: Living in the moment, being "present," is where true happiness lies. Here's good news: Utilizing MOPSI *requires* that you be present. These activities are designed to utilize focus and concentration in order to follow the ever-changing patterns of movement. Don't get me wrong, I am not completely anti-tech, but the danger is that so much "i" stuff tends to disconnect us from ourselves. Since my business is bringing attention to both the body and the brain -- in particular, their connection -- I thought I'd drop some simple, easy trivia about this co-op we inhabit, which you might find interesting.

The neocortex, the "thinking" part of our brain, contains eighty-five percent of the brain's one hundred billion neurons. Although the average adult brain weighs about three pounds, it uses twenty percent of the body's blood and oxygen supply to function. By the way, if the neocortex were opened up and spread out like a map, it would cover 500 square inches of the surface it was lying on. Think about THAT! The carotid artery leaves our heart and carries fresh oxygenated blood directly to our brain. This is a good reason to make sure our "cardiac pump" is strong! When physical activity ceases, the supply of fresh blood and oxygen is diminished.

When this occurs, all the systems and tissues in the body suffer. Even our organs can't function properly, and our cells (the stuff we're made of and think with) die. The ten to twenty billion nerve cells that make up the neocortex are like telephone lines that relay information to other parts of the brain. Don't get confused by all these numbers. I know they may not appear to be adding up, but neurons (the one hundred billion) are made up of nerve cells. They use a pint and a half of blood every sixty seconds, use twenty-five percent of our energy supply, and burn about four hundred calories a day. This is what gives us unlimited ability to learn and relearn new information during our entire lifetime. Calculations of space, force and timing, as well as balance and coordination, take place in one twelve thousandth of a second. We process thoughts at about two to three voltage cycles per second. Brilliant!

Oh, wait, there is one caveat: there must be movement. When we move our bodies, our vestibular system in the inner ear sends a signal to an area in the middle brain that sends another signal to the neo-cortex (our thinking brain) to "wake up and pay attention." Believe it or not, this begins even before we are born, at about five months in utero. Without movement to activate this exchange of signals, we don't take in or retain information from the environment. The signals created by movement allow us to learn, remember, and create. Movement and oxygen are interrelated, so we can put the first two letters of MOPSI together to make MO. MO equals more movement, which equals more oxygen! Speaking of oxygen, the air we breathe is made up of only twenty-one percent oxygen, and seventy-nine, percent nitrogen. If our brain requires twenty percent of the oxygen we breathe, then obviously our ability to breathe deeply and fully is of primary importance. Physical movement is the primary way to *move* that oxygen up to the brain. Here comes MOPSI!

Some time passed before I was ready to write this book. I was still working with individual patients and teaching exercise at Tahoe Forest Hospital. I began this book in 2005, the year I created the *Breathworks for Your Brain* exercise program. Because so much research had occurred since 1998, I took those concepts and created an exercise class I described as "Exercise to Make You Think."

I recently visited a nursing home, where the mother of a friend has gone to live. When I entered the lobby, I saw it was filled with elderly people in wheelchairs, or in chairs -- alone. None of them were conversing, there was no interaction. One woman was holding a huge teddy bear to her chest, her eyes open, but not appearing to *see* anything. She started to push her wheelchair forward, and as she did her slipper started to come off her foot. I went over and asked her if I could help her put it back on. She said "Yes." I placed it back on her foot and pushed her chair close to a gentleman who was staring into space. I knelt down in front of him and asked his name. He looked at me blankly. I asked him again. He muttered something so softly and with such little use of the muscles in his face or mouth, I couldn't catch whether or not he had actually responded.

I turned to the woman in the wheelchair and asked her name. "Mary," she answered. I looked at the gentleman and said, "This is Mary. Tell me your name again." No response. He looked at me with a sad, lost look in his eyes. Then, my friend, whose mother I had come to evaluate, entered the lobby. I walked over to her, overcome with grief at the scene I had just participated in. It has made me passionate about spreading the good news: We do not have to end up like the gentleman without a name!

The secret to prevention of that deterioration can only occur from understanding the connection between our body and our brain: That they are totally dependent on one another and preserving them requires taking the appropriate action. Maintaining focus on a task, while doing a physical activity, produces brain chemicals and neurotransmitters that create and strengthen brain cells that keep our brain working and sharp. (It's the *giving up/giving in* that kills us mentally.) What are the things the body and brain need to stay functioning? As I already mentioned, they are Movement, Oxygenation, Play, Stimulation and Interaction. The combination of these ingredients provides what is necessary for both a body and a brain to stay healthy for as long as possible, precluding genetic, accidental, or disease interference. What makes us remember? (A **whole** bunch of things!) Movement: active movement is vital to brain function; brain function is crucial to movement. Movement is the primary transporter of oxygen throughout the body and, most important, to the brain. You noticed "Play" is included in MOPSI. That's because the inclusion of play into your daily activities boosts everything, from the speed of our thought processes to our immune system.

Let me give you a small, example of MOPSI. I worked with a husband and wife, who were 88 and 89 years old respectively. They were both in good health, but he was in the early stages of dementia. When I was asked to spend some time with him, he was having difficulty remembering his children's names. He was showing signs of aphasia, a condition brought on by any of the following: stroke, brain injury, and dementia. He was having difficulty finding words. He knew what he wanted to say, but couldn't access the word. His reaction was complete frustration and a great deal of fear. He felt as though he were losing his mind. So did his family.

His fear and difficulty in expressing himself had caused him to shut down. He quit talking and pulled deeper into himself. This stately gentleman had had both hips replaced, making it necessary to use a walker for balance and stability. He was about 6'3" and no one had adjusted the walker to fit his tall frame. As a result, he walked hunched over, collapsing his chest, making it difficult for him to breathe deeply when standing or walking. He was practically folding his lungs in half! (Try walking around the house taking small, shallow breaths, and see how far YOU get, before you want to sit down.) On my first visit, the position of the walker got my attention. I lengthened it to allow him to stand up fully. Having been in a bent-over position for months, he still stood that way. I asked, "Were you in the military?" He said, "Yes, I was in the Navy." I said, "Well, stand like the military man you are!" That's all it took. He straightened his back, lifted his chest and stood with the dignity this great guy deserved.

I began to engage him in conversation that required him to tell me his children's names. At first, he couldn't remember and struggled in fear and frustration. As I began asking him general questions, he responded with correct answers, although with some hesitation due to his lack of confidence. We would work for about two hours, simply having a back and forth conversation. I discovered that if I simply let him talk, he struggled with only a word or two, but if I asked him a specific question that put him on the spot, his brain froze up and he couldn't access the word.

I gave him the homework of making a list of the things he wanted to tell me on the next visit. He did that the first few weeks and soon thereafter needed only small reminders. I asked him what he did during the week and he'd relate what he had done with only a slight stumble or so. I said, "Hank, can you see you haven't lost your mind or memory at all? It's still all there. Your ability to retrieve just got weak. Your mental picker-upper, so to speak."

As both his confidence and retrieval system began growing, we started playing word games. I would throw out a word, and he had to say the opposite. Examples: top/bottom; black/white; fast/slow; etc. He was slow at first, but over a few weeks, his ability to find words improved. Another word game consisted of going through the alphabet and saying words as fast as we could think of them. We'd take turns, both starting with "A," then "B," and so on. As with the opposites, his speed of thought improved and increased. Stimulating the language centers in the brain produces visual images (that we may not even realize appear); this, in turn, stimulates the memory retrieval system. It's much like playing Hide & Go Seek.

But back to MOPSI. Let's begin with movement. Hank and Jenny told me they had been great dancers when they were younger (actually, up until the time of the hip replacements) and how they missed dancing. I said, "Let me show you how you can still do it." I had him walk over to a flat-bottomed kitchen chair and sit down. Then, I had Jenny sit in another, facing him so their knees touched. We put on some fabulous jitterbug music, they interlocked their fingers and began to dance.

Jenny, who is still spry and active, tended to lead, pushing and pulling their arms to the beat of the music. It was fast and energetic. They were smiling the whole time. After a couple of weeks of dancing, we started playing ball in the house! We set up three chairs in a triangle formation in the kitchen, and began by bouncing the ball to the person next to us. The key was to keep it going -- no dropping or fumbling the ball. Of course, we all did, but the focus it required to keep it going around was great for the brain.

The second phase was for me to shout out whom to bounce to. This involved major participation by the auditory cortex, an area that seniors use less and less as their hearing decreases. It also required fast response from the motor cortex, another one that is often allowed to get lazy as we age. The processing of the word and then following with the physical action forces the brain to work harder; believe it or not, our brain *wants* to work. It is a task-oriented organ/system, and concentration and focus are one of its favorite and most rewarding tasks. The third phase of the ball-playing was to add a second ball. This sped up the pace considerably, and the energy it took to bounce and then catch the balls (in two different directions) involved larger motor (movement) activity. This strengthens the need for rhythm, another necessary component for the brain; more about that later, when we talk about music.

Because of his double-hip replacements, Hank would need his walker for mobility for the rest of his life. One day, as I was driving over to their house, I began to think about having them dance standing up, the way they used to. When I got there, we put on a wonderful slow song they had loved to dance to "The Night Has a Thousand Eyes." I had them both go to the kitchen, where the floor was smooth and easy to slide on. Hank moved inside his walker a little more and stood up straighter, with Jenny on the outside, facing him. She held onto the walker with him, and they danced all around the kitchen floor. At first, Hank was nervous, and tended to look down. Then, I said, "Hank, look into the eyes of the woman you love."

That was all it took to recapture a romantic memory that had been such an important part of their lives together. It became a part of their lives; spending time with exercise, play, and emotional enrichment, so necessary for a whole body and a whole mind. Sadly, later that year, Hank had a necessary surgery that put him in bed for several weeks. He never fully recovered, and he died early this year. Jenny just turned ninety-one and is still going strong!

Back to this "All Systems Go" idea, the biggest miracle of all is how these systems work together, twenty-four hours a day, for let's say, a person of eighty-eight years. That's 771, 392.00 hours . . . all of it without our having to think about it! The heart keeps beating out its rhythm, pumping the oxygen-rich blood throughout our body at an average of 5 liters a minute (at rest), our breath finding a comfortable pace, both responding to our physical activity, our emotional state and, of course, our lifestyle.

Our gut keeps breaking down our food and moving it along the assembly line, separating the useful stuff from the not so useful; storing the glucose for short term energy, converting the other foods to fatty acids for long term energy, sending the sodium, potassium, magnesium, etc. and the amino acids where they need to go, and using the protein to build anything that needs building or repair. Pretty ingenious! Absolutely as miraculous as Willie Wonka's Chocolate Factory. The "connectedness" is what makes it all work: communication between the 25 trillion blood cells that transport that blood, together with conversation between the 50 trillion or so other cells of tissue and bone. That's basically what it all comes down to: communication.

Consciousness is what sets us humans apart from other living things. I am not referring to the ability to feel emotions. I am talking about our response to those feelings. I'm speaking of the "knowingness," the *feeling-ness* of those emotions and our physical responses that accompany those emotions. The knowing we are feeling anger or anxiety or sadness or joy. Noticing how and where we feel those emotions in our body. Noticing what and where we are receiving sensory signals about the state of our body. Are we too hot, too cold, too itchy? Do my feet hurt? Are my pants too tight?

Consciousness exists because of the communication that is constantly taking place between our body and our brain. They're talking to each other. We are talking to ourselves every minute we are conscious. Our cells are talking to each other by a system of communication referred to as "signal transduction." Normally, we are unaware of this function, but the background knowledge that they are *our* thoughts and feelings, is what gives us our sense of self. Being aware of our body and the millions of sensory messages it is sending every minute is where "consciousness" enters. Being conscious of what our eyes and ears, heart rate, respiratory rate, and body temperature are telling us about our environment is all part of our sense of self. In Buddhist terms, being conscious simply means being awake.

Homeostasis is a term meaning a static, constant and balanced state within the internal environment of the body. That means everything within normal ranges for the individual. The things I listed in the paragraph above, are different for each person, depending on age, gender, size, and genetic makeup. Maintaining homeostasis is only one factor contributing to a healthy, fit, *whole* life. Homeostasis works as a negative feed-back system. As long as everything is in balance, it doesn't have to do anything.

I love to describe homeostasis this way: "If it ain't broke, don't fix it. If it is getting weaker, and in danger of breaking, put demand on it. That will help fix it." Demand creates use; use improves function. Here are a couple of good examples: You work in an office and sit all day at your desk. You've noticed lately that when you go out to take a walk, your legs tire easily. Climbing a hill is difficult. Your legs feel weak. You get short of breath faster than you used to. You're only in your early fifties. This can't be happening yet! But, unfortunately, it can. "Use it or lose it," as the saying goes.

When you're at work, do some Sit to Stand exercises before every break. What's Sit to Stand, you ask? Simply push your chair slightly back from your desk, stand up, and sit down very quickly as many times as you can before you get out of breath. If you can do it eight times, GREAT! Make your next goal to do it ten. If you can only do five or six, work towards eight. If you do this every work day, within two weeks you will notice a huge improvement in your strength, endurance, and breathing when you go for a walk or hike on the weekend.

It works! It's not magic; it is the process of putting demand on several systems, using them and seeing improved function. That's all! So what's the secret to living the healthy life that reaps the desirable benefit of increased energy and a new attitude? One of the secrets is movement. Not exercise, but active movement.

MOPSI presents a change from looking at exercise solely as the means of preventing or managing disease or excess weight. It looks, instead, at movement for movement's sake, for both the body and the brain. Incremental exercise is the name of the game, but not in the newly set standard of ten-minute bouts. I'm talking tiny leg jigglin', foot tappin', shoulder swayin', hip shakin', house walkin' in response to music. Easy, body-gentle fun, even silly movements, just to get the blood and oxygen moving, movement that you can adapt and adjust to fit your physical condition and energy level on any given day. These moves can even be done in bed! Note: If you're going to do them in bed, keep your tummy pulled in to protect your back!

Unfortunately, there is an enormous gap between what the traditional, suggested guidelines for exercise standards are and what many sedentary, obese or frail older adults and seniors are prepared or able to do. Many of you may have been overwhelmed by the prescribed *minimum* twenty minutes a day of aerobic exercise -- three times a week, plus the recommended two days a week of strength training. Although these guidelines are based on sound research and positive results, the sad truth is that this is too much for many older adults and seniors to do at one time.

In my work with individuals with early-stage dementia or Alzheimer's, many also have chronic pain of one sort or another. Some of them have systemic diseases like fibromyalgia or diabetes; some are recovering from cancer or a cardio-vascular event. Many have had a back injury or surgery and still have substantial pain. Most have arthritis. The common denominator is that it hurts to move. Therefore, they don't -- any more than they have to. The other common denominator is that their mental sharpness has lost its edge. They begin to experience more short-term memory loss and difficulty with concentrating and maintaining attention.

Most of them have tried to exercise in the past, but, because they were attempting to meet the requirements that have been accepted as standard, they experienced increased pain, additional injury, or severe fatigue. It's a case of "too much, too soon." Inevitably, they reduce their physical activity to bare minimum, and, in many cases, they even become unable to perform the daily tasks that are necessary to living independently. When you teach someone to chair jiggle or chair dance or play ball, you open a whole world of movement, oxygenation, play, stimulation and interaction: MOPSI! They now have a tool to "clean up their act"!

■ ■ ■

Addendum: Keeping Your Wits About You

How do word games work? What are they? It's any kind of interactive quiz that requires searching your language centers and your memory for answers. I have a sharp brain and an excellent memory, yet this is even challenging for me, *because,* as the quizor, I am retrieving words in a context that isn't normal!

Example: Thinking up words quickly, for the quizee to say the opposite of, or rhyme with, requires pulling single words out of the air. This is not the way the brain usually uses words. We use words in sentences, in context and with a connection to something, whether it is a statement, a question, or an answer. There is usually a "motivator" in a healthy brain, meaning that saying a word is preceded by a visual image within the brain. It does not have to come through the eyes (the visual cortex); it comes from one of the language centers in the left hemisphere of the brain, Wernike's Area. This is the area that creates the image of the word in the context in which it is meant, i.e., the word "hammer" may have two or three (or more) different images: one of the actual tool; one of the use of that tool; and one of someone who is drunk: "Boy, is he hammered!"

I'm going to use my eighty-eight year old as a good example. I tell him I will say a word, and I want him to say the opposite as quickly as possible, i.e., "black." Then he'll say "white." I say "top," and he says "bottom." There is a quirky problem to this method. The brain freezes up under stress. If it feels put on the spot, the non-dominant half shuts down, conserving energy, as in man's primitive stages when confronted with danger. The key is to make it gentle, give all the clues you need to; offer as much as is needed to allow the *quizee* to get the right answer, so the brain can send in the reward: dopamine. This applies to opposites, rhyming, or any other way you play with words.

Here's another bit of brain trivia: the reason word games such as crossword puzzles aren't as effective is because it is important to *say* the words out loud. This involves the second language center in the brain, Broca's Area. Broca's Area is where the phenomes or phonics (the sounds that form the words) are formed. The forming of the words originates from the use of muscles in the face, lips, and tongue, to make the correct sound. Broca's Area is in very close proximity to the basal ganglia, the area of the brain that helps control and coordinate physical movement. It is also where dopamine is produced! The more you say the words, the more you are using the basal ganglia, helping to stimulate the production of dopamine, the brain's reward neurotransmitter. That reward means you will do it more often, because it makes you feel so good. Movement, even when it's only in the face, is important.

Here is another fascinating bit of information. As you may have already guessed, I use music with every activity I do with patients, and I suggest you use it with every activity in this book. The reason . . . *rhythm.* As it turns out, rhythmic activity, whether dancing or bouncing a ball, stimulates Broca's Area and assists in being able to "grab" the word you're trying to think of. Broca's Area is also connected to hand movement . . . AH! Sign language!

p.s. A wonderful exercise for those with Parkinson's, MS, or COPD, is to repeat "Peter Piper Picked a Peck of Pickled Peppers" as loud and with as much exaggerated movement of the face and mouth as possible.

Doing the entire little ditty is great for the memory, but even feeding them one word at a time to repeat places necessary demand on the respiratory system, and the muscles in the face, helping to offset the rigidity that is associated with many neurological disease processes.

■ ■ ■

2

THE TRUTH ABOUT AGING ...
ALIVE & WELL

He sat in his wheelchair in the center of the entrance to the dining room. The noise and preparation for lunch, the background rhythm of the scene, the rattle of silverware, cups and saucers being placed at a different beat, the steady sound of footsteps creating the cadence. People were coming and going all around him. Some young staff, some residents. Although many of them said, "Hello, George." he didn't respond.

What got my attention was his size. He was a big man, dwarfing his wheelchair with his broad shoulders and long legs. Hunched over in his chair, his huge hands were lying listless in his lap, a sad, lost expression in his eyes.

I went over to him, stuck out my hand and said, "Hi, George, I'm Nancy. How are you today?"

Without looking up at me or changing his expression, he said," I'm lonely, that's how. There's no one to talk to around here."

I pulled up a chair and sat down in front of him and took one of his large, age-spotted hands in mine. "I'll talk to you George," I said. "I love to talk."

He didn't raise his head or even acknowledge that I had spoken to him. Since George was not an Alzheimer's patient, there had to be another reason he hadn't responded. I decided to persist.

He was over six feet tall, and by his build it appeared he had been strong at some time in his life. I asked, "How old are you, George?" "I don't remember," he replied. "Seventy-something or other. I was born in 1922."

Pleased that he remembered the year he was born, I said, "George, would you like a drink of water?" He raised his head for the first time and looked at me with clear blue eyes, "Yeah," he said. "I'm thirsty." When I returned with the water, I teased, "You're a little grumpy today, aren't you?" "Yeah," he ventured a small smile, looking back down at his hands. "I am."

Are you stuck in this wheelchair, or can you walk?" I asked.

"I don't know," he said. "I s'pose I could if I tried."

I squeezed his hand. "How long has it been since you tried?"

"I don't know," he said, not looking up. "I don't remember."

This is a picture of the tragedy we are witnessing in our society today, an epidemic of Alzheimer's disease and dementia. Our life expectancy has increased dramatically, but, unfortunately, the demands on both our physical and mental functions have not.

Machines have taken over our physical labors: computers in every size, shape and form are doing our thinking for us. We have become a nation of computer, car, and couch potatoes. If evolutionary adaptation were to adjust to how we are using our bodies, we would become a species of small heads with large ears, with eyes that only operate in two dimension, with arms that don't extend out further than a steering wheel or a key pad, and with cupped hands with oversized thumbs.

As any people-watching location will tell you, bellies and bottoms are getting bigger. The nation's posture is atrocious, chests are concave, backs are getting more rounded and our strides are getting shorter. All this is in response to the lack of function, caused by the lack of use, created by the lack of demand. Technology is *aging* us! How about being able to stand up straight, eyes scanning our surroundings, ears tuning in to the sounds that keep us informed of our relationship to our environment, lean, flexible bodies moving at an instant if necessary, and an alert brain processing all the sensory input.

Both physical and mental fitness is a process rather than a possession. It is a way of life that requires ongoing effort and attention to maintain.

The whole purpose of physical fitness is to allow us to live our lives energetically and full of vibrant good health, so that we may continue to do those things that are meaningful for us and keep us happy and fulfilled. Without brain fitness, that isn't possible. More importantly, even someone confined to a wheelchair can live an energetic, vibrant life if their brain is fully functioning.

Norman Cousins once said, "The tragedy of our lives is *not* that we die. The tragedy of our living is what dies *in us* while we live." My meeting with George was in 1998, the year my first *Breathworks* book was published. George was 76 years old, I was 59. This year I turned 77, and the tragedy of George's physical and mental state still haunts me. It has made me passionate about spreading the good news. We do not have to wind up like George!

What I am offering is not a *new* idea: that brain fitness and body fitness are inextricably tied together, but my approach is new and based on the newest neuroscience research out there. We now know that fitness doesn't have to be work, it can be play. You can look forward to it. It can be bouncing a ball to great music, instead of pounding the treadmill to mindless noise coming off the sound system.

OK, let me back up here. Remember, this is actually a brain-training program -- an actual *training* program. You are going to learn ways to use your eyes, ears, hands, feet, balance, timing, coordination, and spatial analysis all at the same time. You're going to practice short-term memory retrieval over and over again . . . with the things you need to remember continually changing, so the amount of things you need to remember keeps growing. As you keep learning -- and remembering -- your brain and endocrine system release wonderful, *feel-good* chemicals, which not only make you feel happy and good about yourself but also promote the growth and strength of the neural connections within the brain. They are actively keeping brain cells alive instead of letting them die off. Sound intriguing?

I have been teaching exercise and how the muscles work together for over twenty-five years. (Here's something you may not know . . . I didn't start this until I was almost 50!) During most of those years, I followed the prescribed method of teaching: make the cardiovascular workout intense, and the strength work tough. I wanted grunts from extreme effort, not done in a playful spoof on a Sumo wrestler.

Guess what? It's a whole new world. Play is in, exercise that's work is out. Breaking a sweat is still in, but perspiring from the "whole-body" involvement in the activity is what counts. We no longer have to conform to old beliefs about what exercise *should* be. This is *using* the whole body to put demand on the whole brain and *using* the whole brain to put demand on the whole body. This is exercise that's play, and play that's exercise!

And you, my friend, -- the forty, fifty, sixty or seventy-something adult who is still excited about life, or wants to be -- want to be healthy and happy enough to participate in your life *fully*. Well, you also want your brain function, your concentration, your creativity, your cleverness, and your ability to recollect all to remain sound. Think about that word, "recollect" . . . *re-collect*; in other words, *retrieve* information from storage in the brain and bring it "front and center." That is part of what this brain training program is all about, practicing retrieval. That process, done over and over again, using different information, sharpens the short-term memory function. But that is only one facet of it. Let's back up a minute. My fascination with brain function and the body/brain connection began in the mid-1990s. Four things occurred that spurred my interest (and then, passion) for working with the body to affect the brain and vice versa. It's time to tell you a story.

First, my four-year-old granddaughter sustained a closed-head injury, then a stroke, from a catastrophic accident. My son asked me to do some therapeutic work with her, and I began using some of my initial *Breathworks* exercises with her to assist her gaining back movement. As it happened, in May of 1995, America's foremost brain researchers had gathered in Chicago to examine the link between exercise and learning. What they found was that exercise not only creates and strengthens bone, increases muscle mass and strength, it also strengthens the basal ganglia, cerebellum, and the corpus callosum of the brain. In fact, they discovered that aerobic exercise actually created about 60,000 new brain cells every day! There was only one problem . . . these new brain cells didn't live very long. Never mind, the new discovery was very exciting.

It was late in 1998 when I discovered Carla Hannaford's ground-break-ing book, *Smart Moves: Why Learning Is Not All In Your Head.* It introduced an old re-patterning program, Brain Gym, established by Gail and Paul Dennison in the 1970s. Carla's book and the Brain Gym program were the key that unlocked the door to my granddaughter's recovery. As I began to use some of these movements with my granddaughter, I began to see an enormous connection between specific types of movement, focused con-centration, and *looking* at the body part she was working with. That was my first clue that consciously involving the visual cortex (the eyes) had an impact on signals between the body and the brain. It made them stronger!

Jumping ahead a few years . . . I began to use my work with Parkinson's patients and other neurologically-based conditions, i.e., cerebral palsy, multiple sclerosis, stroke, and brain injury. Over the next few years, I stud-ied all the research I could find and used my intuition when working with patients.

In the late 1990s and in early 2000, a new approach to stroke and brain injury was introduced by a group of innovative, pioneering neuroscientists -- *Constraint Induced Therapy.* In a nutshell, it was based on the newest science, revealing the amazing *neuro-plasticity* of the brain. It introduced the news that brain injury and stroke didn't automatically mean permanent loss of function. The approach was to "reframe" how we looked at trauma to the brain.

Instead of believing that all stroke or injury caused the immediate death of brain cells and tissue, they re-defined the original incident as being a state of neural shock . . . a period of time in which function shut down (temporarily) in order to regroup, rest and recover. They offered a ground-breaking idea. During the period of shock, prior to permanent loss of function, *place demand* on the affected limb, *require use* of the affected areas, and you could *regain function.* Brilliant! And it supported the birth of my own burgeoning belief that **increased demand creates increased use, creates increased function,** the basis of the Breathworks For Your Brain exercise classes.

The neuroscientists stated that prior to permanent loss of function, learning to do everything with the non-affected areas of the body and brain *allowed* the eventual permanent loss of function due to *non-use*. The non-use was what resulted in permanent loss of function. Wow! Due to the lack of diagnostic methods to look deeper into the brain, and exercise nature being what it is, we had been trying to *fix* the person (and move them on) by jumping to adaptation therapy; teaching them how to compensate for an unusable right hand and arm, by teaching them to simply use the left . . . *Mistaken approach!* As I said in the Introduction, *"How much you use, determines how much you lose."*

Back to the story. Because I had been fortunate enough to attend the first workshop offered at UC Davis, here in California, I began to apply the method to all the patients I worked with, gently of course, but having them repeat an almost impossible movement repetitively . . . five or six times in a row.

What I observed was that after about five repetitions, it was as though a rusty faucet had just cleared and the water was able to flow. Suddenly, you could see a breakthrough; the signals began to get from the brain to the affected area. Movement that had been spastic and jerky began to smooth out. The longer the repetitions, the smoother the movement . . . up to fatigue. Recognizing when the effort became fatiguing was an important factor. You wanted to stop while the signals were firing evenly. Being consistent with this approach re-built muscle memory -- but as in any fitness or training program, the moment the training ceases for about three days, *de-conditioning* begins.

Demand and use maintain conditioning of any kind. Lack of demand and use allows loss of conditioning. Remember what your mother used to say, "Practice makes perfect." Well, the fact is practice maintains and *increases* skill, ability, and facility -- however you want to say it.

Now, don't get me wrong. Vigorous exercise, sustained aerobic exercise, is still the best way to strengthen your heart and lungs, burn fat, and build muscle and endurance. Many people in their twenties, thirties and forties, even fifties, are still going to be drawn to the bigger is better, more-rather-than-less principles. But that is exercise for the sake of exercise. This is different. This is a method of using your body . . . *movement* to strengthen your neural circuitry, your ability to concentrate, your ability to process and retrieve. In other words, think on your feet or in your chair! Just today in class, we all bounced balls, did heel taps AND repeated our times tables! Now, *that's* using the old noggin! We have arrived at a place where we do not need to follow the masses. What we want to do is to find our own way to that place of self-actualization that Maslow talked about. Is that success? I guess that depends on your definition of success. Is it power and influence? Well, I don't know. You tell me; would you be reading this book if you believed those things would make you happy? What if the concept that physical health, physical and spiritual energy, mental sharpness, and the interest and enthusiasm for life was what motivated you?

Ahhh, we have a match! You are in for both a treat and a surprise. Brain Training exercise can be more fun than you would have believed. First of all we have to establish that the brain(s) basically run the body. You noticed I said brains (plural) because you will learn there are more than just the one sitting on top of your neck. Nevertheless, NOTHING happens without the brains knowing about it, and usually controlling it. You'll learn that we have a head brain, a heart brain, and a gut brain. Intrigued? Sometimes we make poor choices because the head brain isn't doing its job right; nevertheless, some part of it did give the orders. But here's a news bulletin: what we put *into* our body can affect the way our brains work! The good news is that we have the ability to help all three brains work better by the choices we make about our lifestyle. Now, there's a connection for you. Why do we want to know this? Because when your brains decide to quit . . . well, it's pretty much all over.

Here's a good time to introduce you to "Chair Jiggling," a totally silly, very effective way of introducing movement into your life. Here's how it works: you put on some music (that you enjoy) that has a strong beat. Now, here's the cool thing, it doesn't have to be pop, rock and roll, blues, or country music -- the music you usually associate with having a strong beat for dancing. I have done this to Bach, Mozart, Rachmaninoff, and Tchaikovsky. Just envision a conductor leading a symphony orchestra to any classical music. Is he stiff, body quiet, only leading with his hands? I think not! He gets his whole body into it, because the natural desire to move to music or any sustained beat is primitive. We were dancing to the rhythm of sticks being struck together before we were doing agriculture! Sorry for the side bar, but back to jigglin'.

Alright, you've put on some favorite rock or pop song and you're ready to go. Sit in a straight-back, flat-bottom chair, like a kitchen chair. The good news is you can also do this in a wheelchair! Sit so that both feet can be *flat* on the floor, with your back nice and lengthened. In other words, don't slump. Sit like a child who is excitedly waiting for the next surprise. Listen to the music for a minute or two until you hear a repetition of a pattern in the way the music flows. Close your eyes (if you can) and allow your body to move in response to the rhythm of the music. Start with tapping your foot while you tap your hand on your knee; as you begin to relax and *feel* the music, let your shoulders get involved and then, finally, your hips. Keep the heel on the floor, lift your toe and tap to the beat. Alternate your toes, then lift the heel and continue tapping to the beat.

Now you're working the back of your lower leg legs. Let's add the shoulders, just a small movement back and forth, first one shoulder and then the other. Don't be stiff (no one is watching you) but *let* your shoulders move to the music. You may notice that when you start moving your shoulders, you're also moving back and forth on your fanny. You *actively* involve the hips by gently squeezing first one cheek (on your bottom!) and then the other. In my classes, I call this "bun bobbling." Although you may not be aware of it, when you squeeze your fanny, the muscles in the thighs also become engaged. Pretty soon your whole body is movin' and groovin' to the music.

If you were ever a dancer, or wanted to be a dancer, this will be easy. If not, this may take some real effort to keep your inhibitions out of the way. But think of it this way -- if you haven't been getting any regular physical activity that involved the whole body, this could be a matter of life or death! Certainly, of quality of life. The good news is, no one needs to see you do this. If you can sustain your movement for the length of a whole song, you have done something amazing for your body AND for your brain. Oh, one more thing, you can even jiggle in bed. Turn on the radio, or your iPad, find an up-beat tune you love, pull in your tummy and jiggle yourself awake. You'll jump out of bed with a smile and great energy.

So let's take that chair jiggling and make it a little more complex. In renown author and Harvard professor Dr. John Ratey's latest book, *Spark The Revolutionary New Science of Exercise and the Brain,* he says: "[. . .] the more complex the exercise, the better. Compared to rats running on a treadmill, their cohorts who practiced complex motor skills improved brain-derived neurotrophic factor (BDNF) more dramatically, which suggests that growth is happening in the cerebellum." All this means is that there is a brain chemical released in your brain when you're having fun, which actually strengthens, thickens, and protects the actual neurons in your brain, AND speeds up the transmission of synapses (the communication between two neurons.) This chemical, called "Brain-Derived Neurotropic Factor" or, more simply, BDNFs, was discovered in two different studies. One, at the Brain Research Institute in Los Angeles, California, and the other, a co-study between Columbia University of Medicine and the Salk Institute. All the more reason to do the movements suggested in this book!

Begin tapping your right toe to the beat of the music. After 8 taps, start tapping your left heel at the same time and keep them both going. After you've done 8, both at the same time, switch and repeat the pattern, starting with the left toe for 8, then add the right heel. (Here's a safety hint: If you have a bad back, sit on the front of the chair, keep your tummy pulled in, and back lengthened.)

Wow! I bet you feel that in your lower legs, but after you've rested a moment, repeat the whole thing, then repeat both legs in sets of 6, 4, and 2. It sounds (and looks) deceptively simple, but you had to *think* about the exercise as you were doing it. You were doing math and chair dancing at the same time. That's fabulous! When an older adult begins the downward spiral into dementia or Alzheimer's, the ability to care for one's self is one of the first things to go. That is tragic. The good news, even with a genetic predisposition to those diseases, we have the ability to slow down, intercede, or possibly avoid that devastating possibility. It certainly is worth a try.

So what's the secret to living the healthy life that reaps the desirable benefits of increased physical strength and energy, plus an increased ability to process and retrieve information, stay focused and interested on a task? One of the secrets is physical activity. Notice I didn't say exercise, I said physical activity. In other words . . . <u>active movement</u>. Not moving can kill us. We don't have control over our genetic risk factors for disease, nor can we go back and undo all the damage we may have already done by smoking or abusing food and alcohol, but we can affect our health and our future by introducing physical activity, particularly play-based activity, into our lives . . . and *it doesn't matter* if all you have been doing is sitting in front of the TV until now. If you can find an activity that makes you smile at others and laugh at yourself, you have a chance not only to extend your life, but you can make every moment of it worth living.

In June 2003, *The New England Journal of Medicine* reported on The Einstein Study done at Rush Alzheimer's Disease Center, Rush-Presbyterian St. Luke's Medical Center, Chicago, Illinois. They looked at factors that can help ward off or slow down Alzheimer's disease and vascular dementia. The study gave participants a variety of *brain-stimulating* activities: doing puzzles, playing cards, reading and writing, playing board games (including group discussions), and listening to music. They also had them participate in eleven physical activities, such as swimming, riding a bicycle, dancing, etc. Guess what? **The only activity to benefit the brain measurably was dance.** Joseph Verghese, who was the lead researcher, stated that the study revealed that those participants who danced frequently -- three or four times a week -- showed 76 % less incidence of dementia than those who only danced once a week, or less. More good news . . . it's never too late to start!

So, if you haven't been moving until now, that's still OK. It really is never too late to start to improve the quality of your life; and even if it is advised to get 30 minutes of exercise and even break a sweat, you know what . . . something is better than nothing. The predominant evidence is that *disuse*, not the aging process, causes deconditioning. That goes for both the body and the brain. With the exception of those individuals with specific disease processes going on, there is no physiological reason for us to experience early physical deterioration – except inactivity.

What does this mean? It means making the physical activity a positive experience, providing the opportunity to learn a new skill and thereby giving the participant a sense of reward, result in increased neurogenesis (growth of neural cells) and support the production of important neurotransmitters (dopamine, acetylcholine and norepinephrine; the *feel good* brain chemicals that are necessary for learning and memory). Chances are, just doing another crossword puzzle (even if it IS the *New York Times*), isn't going to trigger that amazing sense of accomplishment and pride you will get when you learn something new, discover you can still do something you thought you'd lost the ability to do! Mike Merzenich, founder of The Brain Fitness Program and often referred to as "The father of neuroplasticity" says this: "Getting joy out of what you do is critical to keep doing it." In other words, doing exercise that provides "little flickers of happiness" is the key to pumping up the dopamine system and stimulating improved cognitive function.

Second, and equally as important, is focused attention. Without concentrated attention, information taken in does not register in the brain. Paying attention decreases neural activity in the areas of the brain not involved in focusing on the target of your attention and literally *increases* the size of the area being used. Concert violinists and pianists, as well as chess masters, all show enlarged cortical areas in the brain corresponding to the practicing of a skill demanding intense concentration. Recent studies using primates taught to pay attention to only one signal (as both sound signals and sensory information was sent to their fingers), showed clearly that neuro-plastic changes occurred only in the areas the monkeys were focusing on. No changes occurred in the areas of the unnoticed signals.

MOPSI is based on a simple physical principle: **Increased Demand *creates* Increased Use *creating* Increased Function.** Remember what I said at the beginning of the chapter? It's all related to the need for function. Let me tell you how it works. During the pattern-based exercises, the brain must connect the following: auditory and visual input with processing of the information; planning with anticipation; balance with meter, rhythm and pace; spatial awareness, direction and force; coordination in partner activities; focused attention on where they are in the pattern; short-term memory retrieval of the pattern itself. While this is happening, every nerve and muscle is involved in the coordination of the physical movements. Within the body, oxygenated blood, neurotransmitters, hormones, lymph, as well as cranial-spinal fluid, are moving. The dance/ball playing and strength exercises activate, engage, and integrate the body and the brain simultaneously. These activities override age boundaries, disabilities, depression, and negative self- image, while they are strengthening the heart, lungs, bones, and muscles.

Dance and play allow us to explore our relationship with both our body and with others. These activities create new interoceptive maps within the brain. Interoceptors are *neural sensors* within the body that react and signal when we're thirsty, cold, hungry, or have had a change in blood pressure. For instance, our arteries have a baroreceptor within them, which signals the arteries to open wider or constrict to stabilize blood pressure. Another great example: where a muscle attaches or inserts into bone, there is a sensor called a Golgi Tendon Organ, and its role is to prevent the muscle from being pulled off of the bone. This is most evident when stretching.

By starting your stretch and holding for a count of 20, you will notice the muscle beginning to relax. The GTO signals the muscle that it can relax and allow the stretch. These neural sensors play a huge role in both increased body awareness and in fall prevention. The message here is: *Pay attention to your body*. The fact is, 40 to 60 percent of the fibers within a muscle are sensory nerve fibers. The purpose is to keep you from hurting yourself! Therefore, *notice* the signals your body is sending you: "Slow down, pick up your feet, don't try to lift that heavy box . . ."

The aging brain normally slows down in its processing of information, but, if free from disease, can remain as vital and as good at learning and performing tasks as a young brain. *The biggest change is the decline in our sensory perception and awareness, which is the way we take in most of the information we learn.* As we age, and our vision becomes less sharp, we pay less attention to detail. As our hearing diminishes, we pay less attention to what people are saying and to what's going on around us. Without stimulating input from our eyes and ears, our brain doesn't take in as much information, so we use less of our brain. Paying attention is *crucial* to taking in information. Taking in information is *crucial* to learning!

Movement of our eyes, head, body, and feet stimulates the vestibular system, which plays a crucial role in our development and learning throughout our lives. As we move less, our muscles weaken, our bones become more fragile, and our balance and stability gets poor from lack of use. It's all connected. The health and use of one system is dependent on the health and use of other systems. Movement is necessary, not only to promote the flow of oxygenated blood throughout the body and to the brain, but also to produce acetylcholine, a primary brain chemical for memory and attention. Acetylcholine is a "messenger." When it is released into the muscle fibers, it sets up a chain of events that results in muscle contraction.

Our muscle fibers contain special proteins that stabilize the nerve receptors. These nerve receptors are like "docking stations" for the acetylcholine to go to. Inactivity (lack of muscle contraction) causes a breakdown in the proteins that make these docking stations. Without muscle contraction, you don't produce acetylcholine, and without the proteins, you don't produce the docking stations. Without someplace for the acetylcholine to go, the brain doesn't produce this important brain chemical. It's all interrelated and connected.

The loss of receptor activity reduces the number of signals within the brain, and the loss of use ultimately results in the loss of function. Coordinated movements are particularly important. They stimulate the production of other brain chemicals that stimulate the growth of nerve cells and increase connections.

MOPSI actively uses the eyes, ears, and muscles, specifically targeting the cerebellum and basal ganglion, which are responsible for the organization, timing, control, force, spatial awareness, and speed of our movement. Rhythmic movement allows a fluid interaction between the muscles and the cerebellum and basal ganglia, which, in turn, sends signals to the neocortex (the frontal lobe of our brain) and which organizes our thoughts. It's all connected. Isn't that fabulous!

So, increased use of the body results in increased and improved use of the brain. While you are using the DVD as your training aid for the exercises, *look* at these older adults and seniors ranging in age from their late 60s to well into their 90s. You can see the speed with which they are processing the visual and auditory information I am giving them. The results speak for themselves. What am I really saying? Repeating changing sequences of foot movements (simple tap dancing) with the larger motor demands of bouncing and tossing a ball to a sustained rhythmic pattern of music, requires intense, focused attention on the activity by the participant. (That's you.)

The results are measurable improvements in strength, balance, coordination, space, timing analysis, and visual/auditory awareness. The benefits in cardiovascular and musculoskeletal health are matched by an increase in fine motor activity and reaction time. Let's not forget the most important factor, measurably increased blood flow and oxygen to the brain! Mike Merzenich says, "The discoveries of neuroplasticity will usher in a new brain culture, understanding the need to exercise your brain as you exercise your body." What does this mean? It means that within your everyday life there is opportunity to move. There are ways to turn the activities of daily life into a form that can improve your overall health, prevent or manage disease, and benefit both the quantity and quality of life. Unfortunately, many older adults get the message from almost all advertising that health and fitness equate to a young, hard body, often the result of near starvation diets and hours spent in the gym or running marathons.

Is it possible that there is a more realistic approach to both the visual images and the definition of fit? I'm here to tell you that there is.I realize that may sound so boringly scientific that you want to completely skip this part. What matters is: *eat healthy, balanced meals as much as you can and decide to start moving on a regular basis every day.* You will strengthen and improve both your body and your brain. Simple as that!

This combination creates an *inviting* image of an older adult: an adult at a healthy weight, without the potentially dangerous build-up of fat around the belly, one with good posture and sparkling eyes and an attitude that manifests a continuing enthusiasm for life. That's the image we should be selling, because older adults are what we eventually are all destined to become. Some of us are already there!

In one of my classes there is a couple (he's 89, she just turned 90) who do the class two or three times a week. She was a tap dancer in Hollywood in the early days of the movies. She's tiny but not bent over, thicker around her middle than she used to exercise, but not overweight, and her eyes sparkle with the energy and vitality of a woman fifty years her junior. Her husband is in the early stages of Alzheimer's, yet they both execute the dance steps we do with the joy of doing something they remember well, dancing to music that makes them smile. As they are doing this, they're strengthening their hearts and lungs, as they also strengthen their bones and keep muscle on their limbs. How great to do all that and have fun at the same time! With the predicted average life expectancy increasing to 80 or older, it becomes more and more important that we increase our understanding of how we age, and what we can do to make sure we age *well*.

In *Audacious Aging*, Elite Books, 2009, Deepak Chopra writes, "We are the only creatures on earth who can change our biology by what we think and feel." He goes on to say that we possess the only nervous system that is *aware* of the phenomenon of aging, and because we are aware, we have the ability to influence how that occurs.

What he is referring to is that *what* we believe about *how* we are destined to age, *affects* how we age. What we *believe* about how we are destined to change and age, *impacts* our choices and our behavior and ultimately impacts how we age. What we believe directs the behavior of every cell in our body. If you don't believe that yet, stay tuned, because I intend to share the newest scientific findings on this very subject. It's equally important that we understand some specific scientific facts, if we're to effectively intervene with the normal aging process. Since the purpose of this book is to motivate you to keep your body moving, I believe you need to know *why* – then I'm going to tell you how to start. It's fun, not frightening. It's doable, not impossible to think about . . . and it works!

■ ■ ■

3

BEGINNING OF THE END . . . (WHAT YOU MAY NOT WANT TO KNOW)

Aging is not for sissies. You hear that a lot these days . . . at least I hear it a lot, because I AM aging, my students are, and believe me, it isn't for sissies. We are all suffering from: stiff necks, knees, knuckles and sore joints; thinning skin that bruises or tears at the slightest insult; and the need to find a pair of glasses just to *find* your glasses.

B. F. Skinner, the noted Harvard behaviorist, said: "If you want to know what it's like to get old, smear mud on your glasses, stuff cotton in your ears, put on a pair of thick cotton gloves and a pair of shoes two sizes too big." Although I swore I'd never get that way, I'm afraid at times I have to agree with him. Yet offsetting the physical discomfort and inconvenience is the opportunity to take a lifetime of living and utilize and share that wisdom and experience to improve the quality of life for ourselves and others.

Although actual dementia only occurs in a small percentage of the population (roughly 5%) and the risk of Alzheimer's is actually less once a person reaches the ripe old age of 80, the tragedy occurs when lack of physical movement *and* learning (they're both important!) cause a blurring of sensory awareness, alertness, inquisitiveness, mental flexibility, and humor. One of the saddest symptoms of both Alzheimer's and dementia is the change in personality, often manifesting itself in obstinate behavior and hyper-reactive fear and anxiety. One of the best aspects of MOPSI is the state of pure happiness that the silly exercises and mastery of the patterns of movement bring about.

The brain does age, as does the central nervous system and the rest of our body. Just as the discs between our vertebrae, the lubrication within the joints, as well as our hair and skin thin and dry out, so does our brain. It's all caused by cellular death, a naturally occurring phenomenon that actually begins as early as young adulthood. Within both the spine and the brain, the death of nerve cells results in shrinkage or a decrease in weight and mass.

Some of the loss of nerve cells in the spine, muscles, and other tissues affects the transfer of the signals the body is trying to send to the brain about where our body is in relationship to our surroundings. This results in decreased balance, coordination, and awareness of foot placement, which often result in a fall that can be life altering or life ending. Our sedentary lives contribute to that by not presenting daily activities that challenge our coordination, balance, and reflex response. This is a perfect place to teach you a balance and strength movement. I call it: "The Oil Derrick."

Stand, holding firmly on to either the back of a kitchen chair or a counter top, at your side. Holding on with your left hand, raise your right arm straight up overhead. Simultaneously, lift your right knee to a 90 degree angle, as you bend your right elbow and pull your arm down to your knee. Immediately, bend forward from the hip, extending your right leg straight out in back of you and your right arm straight out in front. Keep them both fully extended (straight) for a count of three. Return to your standing position, pause for a count of three and repeat 3 more times. Then switch and repeat with your left side. You will need to watch the DVD for this one, but it is perfect training for bending over to pick something up off the floor. Keep your eyes fixed on an object straight ahead of you when you are standing, before and after the bend to give your vestibular system time to adjust. Important: **If this move makes you dizzy, do not do it!**

Our grandparents lived in a world that presented challenges at every front. To start, clothing was bulky and stiff, hard to move in and miserable to keep clean on dirt streets and dusty wooden sidewalks. There was no animal control in those days, so just imagine how often your dear grandparents stepped in dog poop and then had to stop and unlace those boots while bending over in those corseted bodies and stiff collars. Every day required significant physical activity just getting dressed; housework and transportation also required large muscle group strength, dexterity, and endurance. Life was full of continual physical activity and was a continual learning experience. It was also much shorter in those days. Ramble around an old cemetery and read the gravestones. People usually died before the age of 70, and every day was challenging. In the evenings when tasks were over, men read, carved wood, or played checkers. Women did needlework or mended socks and patched overalls. There was very little *idle* time, and everything except reading a book was in three dimension . . . the world we were meant to live in.

Yet today, in a world dominated by technological innovations, household and occupational tasks can usually be accomplished with little physical exertion. The motivation for physical fitness is no longer just to have the physical energy to make it through the day, but that we may live integrated, meaningful, satisfying, and joyful lives. In addition to this, persons who are physically fit are less at risk of disease and are better able to function at the peak of their abilities. It naturally follows that someone who is educated about their body is better able to take control of their health. Understanding how the systems are interrelated to each other and the interconnectedness of your functioning on whole-health play an important role in creating healthier lifestyles.

Let's talk a little bit about our bodies so you can see how everything is connected. As early as 1991, the highly respected expert on aging, William Evans, PhD, Professor of Nutrition and Medicine at Tufts University, wrote: "The fact is, we not only can lose up to 50% of our muscle mass with age, we also lose motor units. A motor unit is comprised of a set of muscles and the nerves that signal them to move. A senior in their 70s, who doesn't exercise, loses as much as 20% of the motor units in their thigh, and those motor units are predominately for strength."

In his groundbreaking book *Biomarkers*, he writes that from the age of 30 on, our lean muscle mass begins to decrease a little more than half a pound a year. He labeled this process as *Sacopenia*, coming from the Greek words that describe less flesh. A *New York Times* article, August 30, 2010, released news of new concern from the medical community over this phenomenon. A process that has been going on since the beginning of man's time is now of renewed interest to the scientific and medical world, just like the new interest in the aging brain.

After age 45, this process speeds up so that by 70 an older adult may have lost more than 30% of their muscle. More importantly, they may have replaced that with body fat. Evan's theory was then (as it is now with the newest science on the brain) that disuse or reduction of demand on the systems allow and may even contribute to the loss of cellular life, whether it's muscle tissue and bones or brain cells. (What'd I tell ya?)   I don't mean to depress you, but there's more. To give you a break, let's pause and practice what I'm preaching! Here is a simple, completely portable way of strengthening the muscles in both the front and back of your legs, *anywhere* you are sitting down . . . say, in front of your computer, or in a long and boring meeting at work. You could even do this in an airplane, as long as you explain to the flight attendants you are doing your strength exercises, NOT trying to disrupt the flight. It goes like this:

Sitting on the front part of your seat, make sure your feet are *directly* under your knees, your knees *directly* in front of your hips. Now, simply press down through the bottom of your feet *as though* you were going to rise . . . *but don't*. Hold the press for a moment, then release. If you have any question as to whether this contracts your muscles, place your hands on your thighs so your fingers can squeeze into the outside and inside. Feel the muscles working? You bet your life! Now do this 12 times and I guarantee you will feel fatigue in the muscles. Simple, easy, portable -- and most important -- effective. Is it a brain training exercise? No, but it certainly creates the flow of fresh blood and oxygen, and nourishes the brain! Several years ago guidelines issued by the *Center of Disease Control and the*

American College of Sports Medicine recommended light to moderate physical activities to optimize health. So, the operating word is movement, movement, movement.

Every *system* in the body relies on blood flow and oxygen to function. Our respiratory and circulatory systems, *all* the internal organs, including the reproductive organs, the bladder and kidneys, and the immune system, as well as our muscles and bones, all require a continuous supply of fresh blood and oxygen to be healthy. The most important system of all may be brain function. With the cessation of physical activity, the continuous supply of fresh blood and oxygen is diminished; and guess what, they have even discovered that cerebral (brain) blood vessels can grow as a response to exercise! With decreased or limited blood flow and oxygen, all the systems and tissues in the body suffer, proper organ function is affected, and cells (the stuff we're made of, and *think* with) die. The answer? The more you move the body (the *whole* body), the more blood and oxygen get to where they need to go!

The medical community has known for a long time that life-altering diseases like heart disease, hypertension, diabetes, cancer, and osteoporosis, just to name a few, can be slowed down, arrested, or even avoided by a program of regular exercise. But many non-disease related problems that seniors experience, like poor circulation to the hands and feet, digestive problems and constipation, insomnia, even vision problems, can be significantly improved with light to moderate exercise. Okay, let's take this back to the brain. The increased blood flow and oxygen delivered to the brain as a result of physical activity promotes healthy cognitive functioning. This is not to say that an unsuspected aneurysm can't occur, resulting in loss of function in even a fit, active adult.

But the mental decline that occurs in many older adults, without a specific disease process that is neurologically based, is the result of cessation of movement. Sitting in front of your TV all day, watching game shows, can literally kill you. Research has established that the reduction in mental performance is directly affected by reduction in physical activity -- movement. Just walking is great for the brain. It increases blood flow, oxygen, and even glucose that the brain needs to function. What if there was an easy, fun way to do the same thing without having to leave your house? What if the weather is so foul you can't go out to play golf or ride your bike? What if you work all day and don't live in a neighborhood where walking is practical or safe?

In Chapter One, I introduced you to "Chair Jiggling." You already know how to do that. If you're ready to do something more active, I suggest fast walking around your own house or apartment. Even if it's small, it works. Put on some music (always) and listen for a minute or two until you hear a repetition of a pattern in the way the music flows. You can start by walking in place to the music. How fast the music is, is up to you, but a strong 4/4 beat works best. Here's a secret. When you listen to familiar music that you really like, a part of the brain, the cerebellar vermis activates movement of the head, neck, shoulders, and trunk. Your body *naturally* wants to move to music. Depending on the layout and the space you have to work with, pick a route that you can walk in a straight line to a point where you circle around something (like a dining room table) or just walk into your kitchen, turn around and head back. You keep repeating this process for the length of one whole song, usually about 3 1/2 to 4 minutes long. If you're playing a CD that has several songs on it, when the new song begins, reverse your direction and do it again. You can keep this up for as long as you want. Bend your elbows, and pump your arms while you're walking, to make it a whole-body movement. Make sure you are fully using your feet. As we age, our ankles tend to get both stiff and weak, a major concern for older adults who resort to the "senior shuffle" because they don't have the ability to roll through their foot from heel to toe as a normal step should be. As we get older, the tendons in the top and bottom of our feet shorten and get tight (as do our calf muscles!) and have a big impact on our ability to walk on uneven surfaces. Have you noticed that?

Don't be stiff, no one is watching you, so let your whole body move to the music. You may notice that when you start moving your shoulders, you're sort of moving back and forth on your fanny too. You *actively* involve the hips by gently squeezing first one cheek (on your bottom!) and then the other. In my classes, I call this "bun bobbling." Although you may not be aware of it, when you squeeze your fanny, the muscles in the thighs also become engaged. Pretty soon your whole body is movin' and groovin' to the music. This may take some real effort to keep your inhibitions out of the way. But think of it this way. f you haven't been getting any regular physical activity that involved the whole body, this could be a matter of life or death! Certainly of quality of life, and the good news is, before long you may find a park, or a school track where you can safely take your walking outside! Sunshine and fresh air will double the benefits. Walking is weight bearing and if possible we want as much of our physical activity to involve weight bearing because that is so important to keep those bones strong.

If you can sustain your movement for twenty minutes or more, you have done something amazing for your body AND your brain. More about that later, and remember, life is all about choices. To do this activity is *your* choice, the music you walk to is *your* choice, to try something new that could change your life for the better is *your* choice; and guess what, in the next chapter, we're going to start actually dancing; AND you can do this with a partner, even if they are wheelchair bound. The really good news is that almost *anyone* can find a way to integrate movement into their life. You can jiggle your body to music even if you're confined to bed. So be courageous, be adventurous! Give it a try and just see how you feel. I promise, you won't be sorry!

Stand up and put your music back on -- something you will *really* want to move to, like Doobie Brothers, or Fleetwood Mac. If you're younger, any pop or Country Rock will do. Start to tap that foot. (Remember to use the DVD as an aid if you're unsure how to start!) If you're like me, you won't be able to contain the movement of your foot for long. You'll find your shoulders *automatically* get into it, and then your hips ... *blood and oxygen, blood and oxygen.* Many of the changes that we believe are caused by aging are in reality caused by inactivity and poor nutritional habits. What it boils down to is that neither a fixed process of cellular degeneration, or our genetics, affects our physicality in our mature years as much as our choices.

A 1999 *Mayo Clinic Health Letter* stated, "Exercise is the single most important anti-aging measure anyone can follow, regardless of age. To help your body stay young, try to get at least 30 minutes of exercise a day. I'm changing that to say "full- body movement," and even 15 minutes is a great way to start! Now realistically, we know that isn't always possible. Not only do busy schedules, children, elderly parents and just everyday life interfere with the best of plans, what about the millions of older adults out there who have too much weight on them, limited income, little motivation or a disease process like diabetes, Parkinson's, arthritis, etc. that stand in the way of their achieving that difficult goal of 20 to 30 minutes a day. The key is incrementally. Ten minutes at a time, all through the day. Your energy level will increase triple fold. Speaking of increased energy: Here is an exercise that will feel like a workout while you're doing it, but you'll feel energized when you're done.

In your office, riding in a car or RV (while someone else is driving), or in your hotel room: Sit on a flat-bottomed chair with your knees hip-width apart and your feet directly under your knees. Bend your elbows and tuck them into your sides with your palms at chest level and facing forward. Push your arms out directly in front of you (fingers are facing up), then pull back to your chest and push them up over your head. Initially, you just do single pushes: out-in/up-down. It will increase your respiratory workout, if you say, "Out-In/Up-Down," as you do the moves.

Now do doubles, that's two out and in, two up and down. Go back to singles and repeat 2x, then do the doubles 2x. Repeat this combination 4x. Then move up to sets of 3s. Repeat 4x. Finally, do sets of 4, and after repeating 4x, begin to work your way back down (3s, 2s, and singles). This is a real workout for your heart, lungs, and arms. You will definitely feel it when you're done. But what better way to spark up your brain when you've been mindlessly sitting at your computer or riding in a car for several hours. At work, grab yourself a partner and do the exercise with them. Suddenly it's interactive! Change roles with the driver, and let them get a brain boost while you drive. You can't go wrong with this one. You're exercising, remembering and doing math all at the same time. Wahoo!

The fact is, older adults, even *very* old adults, retain the capacity to adapt to increased levels of activity. In laymen's terms this means that our physical strength, energy, and endurance are affected by how strong our bones are, how much muscle we have, how we fuel our bodies, and how we spend our time, even what we think about. It's all connected. *Mopsi* offers simple, fun, effective ways of introducing exercise and active movement into your life that will benefit your brain as much as they benefit your body! Research has now proven that older men and women can achieve the same strength gains as a 28 year old can, as a result of resistance training. Here's another exercise that utilizes multiple muscles at the same time. Even though it is a "pretending to" exercise, it's effective because of the intensity of the muscle contractions as you do it.

Rope Climbing

Stand with your legs hip-width apart, tummy pulled in, back long. Imagine a rope attached on the ceiling of a high school gym. Your goal is to climb that rope, by pulling your body up the rope hand over hand. Reach your right hand up and pretend to grasp the rope. You will make your first pull as you go into a half-squat position. Now, reach up with your left hand and pull your body weight up and you raise yourself up with your legs. Repeat, reaching with the right hand, pulling as though you were lifting your body weight; as you lower into your half-squat, grasp the make-believe rope with your left hand and pull yourself up the rope, raising your weight with your legs as you pull. Repeat this 4x. When you are able, increase to 6x. Remember to *breathe* throughout the exercise.

■ ■ ■

4

TAKING THE NECESSARY STEPS . . .
THE MIRACLE-GRO OF DANCE

One of the first movies I saw as a little girl was *The Red Shoes*. I remember being captivated by the grace and beauty of Moira Shearer as she played out the tragic heroine in Hans Christian Andersen's story. From that moment on, I wanted to be a ballerina. Although that was a flight of fancy that never happened, it stayed cocooned in the deepest recesses of my heart until just about ten years ago. I'm going to tell you a story about how our focused *intention* and *attention* can bring about miraculous changes.

Almost ten years ago we built an Appalachia Log home. That means square logs instead of round, which is western style. My husband was born in North Carolina and grew up seeing these weathered barns and cabins around the country. They are replicas of what the early colonists built when they arrived here from England, Scotland, and Ireland. Most of the settlers to that area were of Celtic origins, and so the music that developed in that region had a decidedly Celtic sound. It's foot stompin', clogging ~~ *Fast* ~~ tap dancin' music.

Just about the time we built the house, Michael Flatley's *River Dance* hit the stage. Irish dance was all the rage. The movie, *Cold Mountain*, came straight out of North Carolina. Being of Scots-Irish descent myself, and with a big imagination, I thought how much fun it would be to have authentic music playing in our Appalachian house. I began to tap my feet. Having watched the *River Dance* video so many times, I knew what the dancing looked like. I found myself making up little combinations of steps to do to the music. The problem was, I couldn't remember the combinations, or the order I did them in, or how many of each step.

I was both horrified at my inability to retain the sequences and frustrated that I couldn't create an actual little dance. I began to really work at the process. I would put together about four steps, say them out loud as I did them, and repeat them over and over until I got it. Then I'd make up four more, do the same thing and then add them together, repeating the process of saying them out loud and repeating the sequences until I got it.

I wasn't obsessed about it, but I was determined. As a result, I focused my attention when I was doing it. I stayed focused until I got the steps down. I didn't know it, but the birth of the "Breathworks For Your Brain" exercises was occurring. I now teach these original step combinations in my classes, making up new ones often. Not only do I remember them, so do my students as they apply their concentration on *capturing* the sequences. Then practice their *recall* skills as we dance in the class. Remember what I said in the chapter on the brain: "Demand creates use. Use creates function."

How does this relate to brain function and short term memory? When I first started this process, I was just like any other 66 year old. Whenever I walked upstairs with a purpose in mind, by the time I got up there I would forget what I had gone for by the time I got there. Try as I might, the purpose wouldn't return until I had gone back downstairs, necessitating another trip back up the stairs. I *always* had to look up phone numbers, and my retention of people's names was getting poorer and poorer (a common complaint of most adults over 60). I'll come back to this story in a minute.

At about the same time, the neuroscience community was sharing some developments in treating Parkinson's disease. They had found that teaching patients the tango affects the tremors and balance instability that many Parkinson's patients experience. I had been working with Parkinson's patients since 1997 and had discovered on my own that repeating patterns of movement had a direct impact on the tremors and balance issues. I would take my boom box with me, put on some Big Band music and have the patient dance while holding onto a chair or counter for support. It not only affected the physical symptoms, it also seemed to energize them mentally and help the fatigue and malaise that many patients experience. Before we go any further, let's do a little dancing and see what you experience yourself!

Put on some favorite dancing music. Personally, I love Glenn Miller's "In the Mood" for its great beat. If you have balance issues, stand, holding onto your chair or counter for support, and just start stepping side to side in small, quick steps. Use the DVD to see how I do it. You can do it with me. We're going to start with a simple 1-2-3-tap step. That's exactly what it is -- you make three small steps in place (like a small march), then tap your toe. The tap automatically shifts your weight to cause you to start on the other foot. You wind up doing a little dance with both feet: 1-2-3-tap, 1-2-3-tap (you can tap either your toe or your heel, it doesn't matter). Keep doing that and letting yourself *feel* what it's like to move your body in time to the music.

When I'm teaching my classes, I've noticed that the repeating of the patterns seems to be the key to the retrieval of the steps. Doing sets of four steps, followed by sets of two steps that I am cueing with my voice and hand signals. I do them enough time for their motor cortex to create the muscle memory. When I can tell the students have the steps, I create a new pattern. It's an add-on process, but never predictable. I don't always do them in the same order, I mix and match in order for them to have to use their retrieval skills. The result is an improvement in their short term memory.

One of the biggest challenges for seniors is moving their feet fast. When I first started teaching my current group, one of the students (who has now been with me for eight years) said, "I can't move that fast." Let me tell you, she *is* moving her feet as fast as I am, and other students in their late 80s are doing the same. She learned that her body and her brain are still capable of processing information at lightning speed. In my classes, 86 and 87 year olds are dancing along with people in their late 50s and 60s.

There are tricks to this. One of them is to make the moves small. When you feel more confident, you can make them bigger. Keeping the moves, both feet and arms, small and close to the body is the way to complete them safely. These elderly seniors are not only moving their feet fast, they're doing complex moves that challenge their balance. They're doing grapevines, box steps, Cha Chas that require moving backwards and forward, crossing one foot over the other. The purpose, of course, *is learning to know where their feet are.* In other words, knowing where they are in relation to the surface they're on. It's all fall prevention and recovery activity, but the main attraction is the fun -- and the great feeling of accomplishment when they master the footwork.

Let's add another easy step to create a combination. Step side to side four times. As you bring your feet together, touch the toe of the following leg, then step back the other direction with it. You don't actually put your full weight on the second step until you're done with the sequence, so it's Step touch, Step touch, Step touch, Step touch. Look at the DVD to understand what I am describing. As you become more confident, you can make your side step bigger, but for now a small step will do. Our eventual goal is full range of motion.

Now you're ready to put the steps together, so it's *1-2-3-tap, 1-2-3-tap, step touch, step touch, step touch, step touch.* Say this out loud as you keep repeating that combination of steps to the music. You have just completed an actual dance. If you only did those two moves, you've given yourself a good little burst of exercise.

When you're ready to put some feeling into it (because you're actually enjoying yourself!), simply allow your shoulders and arms to do whatever you feel like doing. The key is not to be rigid or stiff. Let your body flow to the rhythm of the music, letting your imagination and memory carry you back to a time you may have done this before. One of my students, who is 86 (soon to be 87) said, "It feels good to cut loose."

Here's where the "Miracle-Gro" comes in. If you were to sustain those two dance steps for the length of one whole song, like "In the Mood," or "Pennsylvania 6-5000," you would have generated brain-derived neurotropic factor, the remarkable brain chemical that is produced when we learn something new, complex, and involves active movement (exercise) that we want to do. The wanting to do it is crucial. BDNFs are not produced when you are made to do something. The desire to do it is part of the miracle . . *voluntary exercise or active movement,* and the more complex the activity we are learning, the more BDNFs are produced. The BDNF thickens, strengthens, and lengthens neurons in the brain, so that the speed of signals between neurons is increased. It feeds the neurons, like Miracle-Gro feeds your plants.

According to Jaak Panksepp, a renowned senior researcher in the science of play, BDNFs stimulate nerve growth in our emotional brain, where our memory is initially housed, and in the prefrontal cortex, where we make executive decisions.

In other words, our brain function is improved by playing -- and dance is play, no matter how you look at it. In the book, *Play,* written by Stuart Brown, MD, psychiatrist and respected clinical researcher, Dr. Brown describes the properties of *play* as: done for its own sake, voluntary, instinctual in nature, providing a sense of timelessness; it stimulates improvisation, reduces self-consciousness, and creates a desire to continue doing it -- because it's fun!

Sound like dance? It is! Dance is one of the most *playful* things you can do. In my classes, we *play* at being Irish dancers, flamenco dancers, line dancers and disco dancers. We play at ice skating, climbing ropes, pulling in anchors, polishing cars, washing windows, and being Sumo warriors. It's all pretending, playing-like, imagining, but it creates a sense of fun that is not usually associated with exercise. We combine these imaginary activities into dance steps and therefore raise the heart rate, increase the respiratory rate, pump the muscles full of fresh blood and oxygen and flood the brain with the same necessary nutrients. We create Miracle-Gro for the brain and improve our concentration and recall skill by dancing and playing. Before we increase our repertoire of dance steps, let's talk about the importance of play to the brain.

Play exists in every aspect of the animal kingdom. From polar bears to hummingbirds. Whether on land, in the sea, or in the air, mammals and birds, even octopuses, have been observed "playing around" with objects on the ocean floor. With other behaviors, responses and *consistent* states of being have made adaptive evolutionary changes to deal with ever-changing, unique challenges. It appears that play *plays* a role in survival, otherwise it would have been eliminated. All baby animals play with each other: wrestling, tussling, pretending to bite, playing tag and jumping on top of each other. They are practicing their hunting and survival skills.

Think about our Neanderthal ancestors who made flutes from wood and bone, sat around their fires clacking their sticks to a rhythmic beat, dancing. They were having fun, playing with tools that would also serve a purpose in the development of the first language. The flute gave them the ability to make a noise for warning of danger, or to scare away a predator or blow sweet notes to woo a mate. Play has always existed. A reasonable theory is that it developed (as it does in animals) for a purpose: practice for skills they would need in the constantly changing environment. Playing, whether verbal or physical, offers the opportunity to learn "give and take," very necessary in our social world. It teaches boundaries, what Daniel Goleman calls *emotional intelligence*, the ability to read others emotional response to the game, whatever it is. Makes sense to me!

Let's start with a simple Cha Cha step. Now, a normal cha cha has the lead step start on one side at a time, say with your *right* foot. You take a step forward, then step back next to your left foot, then do three fast steps in place. You begin again with your left foot forward and repeat the sequence. You keep repeating this sequence of steps until you get it. Then ... you're going to pause and repeat the whole thing starting with the left foot first. You definitely need to look at the DVD for this one. Even if you know how to dance the cha cha -- but this is a little too fast for you -- here's a slower version of the same thing that will still give your legs a good workout:

Just start with your step forward with the right foot, lifting the left leg (in back) just slightly off the floor. Then step in back of your left foot and slightly lift your front right foot. Repeat this back and forth 4x, then on the last step, bring your feet together, pause, and begin again starting with the left foot.

If you need to, put on the cha cha sequence on the DVD and do your best to follow along. Remember, it is not important that you get it right the first time. This is a learning experience for a good reason, to make your brain work and remember. Speaking of remembering, one particular activity that creates BDNFs (Brain-derived Neurotropic Factor) is the complexity of what you are learning. Complex activity requires rapt attention, another crucial factor in learning and remembering, no matter how old you are. Here's a great story to prove that:

Yesterday, a woman whom I hadn't seen in five years came to do my class. She had faithfully done my Breathworks For Your Brain classes for several years. She had lost her husband in the meantime, had some minor health issues, but still looked great and fit. She had always been an avid hiker and played tennis. I asked her how old she was. She said she was 87. My mouth must have dropped open when she said, "I thought I was about ten years older than you."

When I began the class, I used the music and the warm-up moves I had done years before. She simply did them . . . and all the rest of the moves, as though she had never been gone. She even did the Cha Cha sequence perfectly that I had described earlier. As I watched her, I said, "That, my dear, is muscle memory. Your body still remembers these moves." That was exactly what it was, and how marvelous to observe it in a healthy, fit 87 year old!

In a completely different "primitive" aspect, our first movements as infants were expressions of emotion: excitement, happiness, discomfort, and irritation are all expressed in movements of arms, legs and torso, by an infant who has not yet developed the use of language. Body language is how they communicate what they feel. Dance is also one of the most primitive of all forms of expression, communication and celebration. Carvings of groups dancing have been found dating back more than 9,000 years; dancing appears to have been part of the earliest agriculture rituals. They danced for rain, for good crops and in celebration of a good harvest.

When we dance as adults, we can reconnect with that earliest part of ourselves that expressed joy with our bodies, just as children do. Music *moves* us. The brain processes the music that we enjoy in the pleasure centers. The same areas that are involved in our response to food and sex. Making music predates dancing, and even agriculture. Archeologists have found music instruments, carved from the bones and horns of animals, as old as 53,000 years ago.

It appears our Neanderthal ancestors may have soothed themselves with sweet-sounding flute music as they sat around their fires at night. Listening and responding to music is ancient; that is part of what makes it such a powerful tool for the brain. Music and dancing both benefit the body. When you use music with a clear rhythmic beat, the diverse areas of the brain involved in the completion and efficiency of tasks are synchronized, and function is improved. Remember chair jiggling? Coordinating movement of the neck, torso and hips requires thousands of neural signals to multiple areas of the body simultaneously. Think how complex that is, and while you're giving your brain that boost, your muscles are getting used, pumping fresh blood and oxygen from the heart, all through the body, to those muscles, up to your brain and back to the heart. Pretty mind-boggling, isn't it? This is where I finish my story about my own brain changes from this dancing process.

My experience is certainly more dramatic than those of my students. Not only do I teach this five times a week, I'm making up new sequences (and practicing) all the time. Suddenly I began to realize that I was developing a much better memory of telephone numbers . . . even ones I only call a few times a year -- my dentist, my orthopedist, my car repair guy, certainly my students. I'd think about the number I needed to remember, picture it in my head, and BOOM, there it was!

So I began to practice on the process of remembering names. When a new student would come to class, or I'd be introduced to someone, I'd look closely at their face and repeat their name out loud several times. I would try to identify one outstanding feature of their face, i.e., bright blue eyes, or dark eyebrows. My focus and intention were fierce. I was determined to remember. Guess what? I did, and continue to do so. Once it's in there, I don't lose it . . . as long as I keep practicing (the operating word) the process. Looking (or practicing), focusing, and saying it out loud. Six years ago, I took a standardized memory test. According to my neuro-feedback therapist consultant, my scores were "off the charts," meaning AMAZING for a 71 year old.

Now let's address chair dancing. What in the world is that? Well, it's getting all the benefits of regular dancing, but doing it in a chair -- even a wheelchair. If you are in a wheelchair, but are still able to move your feet, then open the foot pedals to the side, so your feet can touch the floor. If it's just the front half of your foot, it will still work. In a regular chair, sit so that both your feet are flat on the floor. Pull your tummy in, lengthen your spine and we're ready to go. We'll start with the *1-2-3-tap, 1-2-3-tap*. As soon as you hear the beat of the music (1-2-3-4, 1-2-3-4 and so on), begin to do the steps to the music.

It doesn't matter where you jump in-in the song, but wait for the first beat of the 4/4 pattern. As you will see, that step allows you to start the sequence with the opposite foot each time after the tap. When you put that foot back down, it becomes the first beat of the next 1-2-3-4, so your tap is always on the fourth beat and with the opposite foot. Think of it this way: Right-left-right-tap, Left-right-left-tap, Right-left-right-tap and so on.

The same concept applies to the step together-step together also. The biggest difference is that the steps are small. Keep them within the width of the chair legs. To make it interesting, alternate four 1-2-3-tap, with four step together. Just keep repeating those patterns for the length of one whole song. That's about three and a half minutes. If you keep it up for five minutes, you've just done fifteen minutes of dancing, either standing or sitting. Hallelujah!!! Okay, so how do you turn this into *whole-body* movement? The easiest way is to pump your arms, (bent elbow) back and forth opposite to the foot that is stepping. That is called contralateral movement, and allows both sides of the brain (hemispheres) to work at one time. It also becomes a powerful "whole-body" exercise or movement, putting demand on the heart to pump more blood with each stroke in order to push it from the heart, all the way through the body (including the brain), and back to the heart again every minute. The pumping of the arms increases your breathing rate as well as your heart rate, so this is one of the BEST methods of avoiding congestive heart failure as we age.

If you can sustain your movement for the length of one whole song, you have done something *amazing* for yourself, and it was your choice. Remember, life is all about choices. To do this activity is your choice, the music is your choice, and to do something new that could change your life for the better is your choice! Be courageous, be adventurous ... give it a try, and see how you feel. You won't be sorry, I promise.

Let's concentrate on the arms for a while. A very simple, silly, and effective way to exercise the arms is to play "Conduct the Music." It is a great upper body exercise, and also works both sides of the brain at the same time. This time, put on some Mozart or Beethoven or Bach -- whatever kind of classical music you enjoy -- but it should be fairly active or *"Allegro"* in musical terms.

Lift both arms up to a level between your waist and shoulders -- about chest height. Hold them out wide, like you were going to hug a roly-poly uncle. When the music starts, begin to move your arms in and out, crossing them in front of your chest; when you come back to center, lift your arms a little higher at the completion of the move before you change directions. If this is unclear, watch it in the video. Now, here's the catch -- alternate the wrist on top each time you cross them. That means you have to be paying close attention to your body as you're doing this!

If you have watched symphonic conductors on television or been fortunate enough to have attended a symphony, you know how wild conductors can be. The more powerful the music, the wilder their movements. If you feel completely unsure about this, put in the DVD, go to Conduct the Music, and follow along. If you want to make yourself laugh, do this in front of a mirror. It is wonderfully silly!

A word of caution: there is no *right* way to do this, but there is a *wrong* way. Making the moves too big can overly stress your shoulders. Keep the moves medium size when you first start. The moves will use your muscles and your joints in all the directions they can go; so do some moves in and out, some up and down. If you have had problems with your shoulders due to injury or surgery, don't move in ANY direction causing pain. Your arms will tire quickly if you do this for the whole song. A couple of minutes is fine to start. You'll feel your heart rate increase and you'll be breathing a little harder. That's what we want, but remember we're just starting here. *Don't overdo!*

Do you remember "Peas Porridge Hot" from when you were a little kid or had children of your own? It's a wonderful child's game of hand movements to a song that follows a pattern. They're rhythmic, active and silly -- all the best components of brain-based exercise. They are also a great way to do "Hand-Dancing." "What is Hand-Dancing?" you ask. Good Question. It is simply another physical way to keep time to the music and have fun!

First of all, I guess I better tell you the words to the little song. It goes like this:

> *Peas porridge hot,*
> *Peas porridge cold,*
> *Peas porridge in the pot,*
> *Nine days old;*
> *Some like it hot,*
> *Some like it cold,*
> *Some like it in the pot,*
> *Nine days old.*

By adding an extra clap after each of the specific hand movements to the words, you give it a 4/4 rhythm. Example: Peas porridge hot, *clap*, Peas porridge cold, *clap*, and so on and so on. If you aren't familiar with the childhood game, Peas porridge hot, here's a description. You can also watch it on the DVD.

It requires two people facing each other to play it as a game, which I'll describe first: The first two phrases have three words: Peas porridge hot, Peas porridge cold.

Each word has a hand action: Peas -- you slap your legs -- porridge -- you clap your hands together in front of you -- hot -- you and your play mate clap your hands together between the two of you. Now, this is where I ADD the extra clap to make it 4/4 time. So you clap your own hands together and then repeat the whole sequence of legs clap, hands clap, and together clap for the word cold, and then end with the extra clap.

Now you're ready for the more complex hand moves. The next phrase is: "Peas porridge in the pot nine days old." More words ... more moves. After the leg slap and the hand clap on Peas porridge, you and your partner clap each other's hand *diagonally* for the phrase "In the pot, nine days -- on "old" -- you and your partner clap your hands together again in front of the two of you.

The rest of it is simply a repetition of the exact same moves to the last phrases. It is silly, you make mistakes, and ultimately laugh and laugh through the whole game. Not only is it fun, but if you stand far enough from your partner, you are both having to reach your arms out to make contact. You can increase your reach and your heart rate by reaching up high when you do the diagonal hand claps with your partner. The reason? Because the higher you lift your arms, the harder your heart has to work. The faster you do it, the harder your respiratory system has to work -- both of these things are a major way to avoid congestive heart failure, which takes many seniors in their late 80s and 90s.

You ask: What makes you think an 80 or 90 year old can even do this? Because I still work with and teach them. I worked three years with an 89 year old and her 91-year-old husband. I worked once a week with them until she was 92 and he was 94 years old. He just got tired of exercising and wanted to sit and watch golf on TV. His choice was perfectly under-standable. He is a Pearl Harbor survivor and did his share of hard work. His spunky wife still gets up and does the exercises I taught them before she gets dressed for the day. She can still get him to do "Peas Porridge" with her!

Like everything else in our bodies, our muscles are made up of indi-vidual cells. Without physical activity, we lose almost 30% of our muscle cells by the time we are 70, and the cells that are left *get smaller!* The smaller the cell, the less power the muscle has to contract. The result is decreased muscular strength. There is also a decrease in the mineral content of our bones. This makes older bones more brittle and more susceptible to break from a fall.

Here's an interesting little story. One of my students, a man in his mid-seventies, who appears to be fit (He's done the class for over a year.), caught his new tennis shoe on the rug two weeks ago and fell onto his side. It looked like a simple fall, nothing drastic or too hard. He got to his feet and sat out the rest of the class. He has asthma, is on Pregnazone, and has red hair and fair skin . . . a classic candidate for osteoporosis. On his way home he had pain when breathing, so he went straight to his doctor. They took x-rays and guess what? The doctor said, "Your bones don't look very good! You've cracked a couple of ribs!"

This was a huge wake-up call. Except for class, he sat all day and worked on his music for the church choir. Just doing the class was not enough. He began to get up every hour and walk for 15 minutes around his house, his yard, or his block. The result? He began to feel better and stronger all over and found he had more endurance than when he was just exercising for an hour, twice a week.

Movement . . . movement . . . movement. That's what it takes.

The major cause of death in the frail elderly is what happens following broken bones as a result of a fall. Fractures of the hip will ultimately end in death 15% of the time, and half of those will require long-term care. Most seniors who break a hip after the age of 80 never return home from the hospital. It's a no-win proposition; something as benign as an accidental fall can have life-altering effects on a whole family.

Another story: I taught an 88-year-old woman who had done the class faithfully for two years. She took a misstep in her apartment, but caught herself before she fell. She recovered but pulled something in her groin, which made weight-bearing uncomfortable. She was hesitant to put her full weight on her leg and took a couple of weeks off from class. I had her ice it and gave her some gentle stretches to do. After returning to class, she began doing most of the foot patterns sitting down. After class she confided to me that her self-confidence had been really affected by the unsteadiness of her leg. This is often the beginning of the end for many seniors. Once they lose their confidence, they quit moving altogether, and it's all down-hill from there. Don't let that happen to you! Look at the Fall Recovery exercises on the DVD and do them. Hold onto a chair, or do the moves be-tween them. You'll experience how practicing concentration on *where* you place your foot strengthens your legs as well as the neural circuitry from the muscles to your brain. Your sense of confidence will increase because of your increased awareness of where you are in the space around you.

■ ■ ■

5

THE KNEE BONE'S CONNECTED
TO THE ...

Our whole system is interdependent. When one system is weak, the others are affected. You wear a pair of broken down shoes, or high heels, and your back hurts. You use your arms painting high cupboards or hanging curtains all day … your neck hurts. Hamstrings that are too tight invariably lead to back problems, even neck problems. Poor posture can make your feet hurt. It's all connected.

The fact is, the muscles and tendons in your lower legs and the bottom of your feet are ultimately connected to the small muscles in the neck and at the base of the skull. Next time you lie on your back to stretch your hamstrings, flex your foot and feel your head pull back. If you tuck your chin, you'll get a better stretch in the back of the leg. It's all connected. This book is about treating the body as a whole, not just some of the parts. In fact, this book is about "the sum of the parts." I believe the most effective way to do this is to see just how the *whole body* works together to support itself.

Every muscle in the body moves something. That's what muscle does as it contracts: it pulls. There are three types of muscle tissue: smooth muscle, which is involved in movement inside the body (as in the intestines, the bladder, the uterus, etc.); cardiac muscle, which contains an electrical circuitry of its own, runs the pumping of blood into and out of the heart, creating our heartbeat; and skeletal muscle, which is the way we pull bones together to produce external movement. Both smooth muscle and cardiac muscle are *involuntary*. That simply means we don't have to think about moving the food we eat along our digestive tract, nor do we have to remember to tell our heart to keep the blood moving.

Okay, now that we've talked about the cardiac muscle and the smooth muscle in the gut, let's talk about the fact that both the heart and the gut have a brain. Surprised? Amazed? Skeptical? Well, they do, and here is the nitty-gritty on them. In 1990, the science of neurocardiology emerged and has been growing ever since. We now know that the heart has 40,000 nerve cells called baroreceptors. It has its own network of neurotransmitters, proteins, and its own support system. It has very sophisticated abilities to compute or think. The *heart brain* acts independently of our head. The average healthy heart beats about 100,000 times a day. In a fetus, the heart develops before either the nervous system or the thinking brain have developed. The electrical signal and its information are pulsed to every cell of the body with every heartbeat. Every heartbeat sends a chemical messenger throughout the body: atrial peptide. This is a primary driver of our behavior, and therefore affects outcomes. So, listen to your heart and take care of it!

Here comes some more fascinating information: there is a brain, a deep, complex nervous system that lies deep in your gut. It contains more nerve cells than the spinal cord or all the rest of the peripheral nervous system and has 100 million nerve cells in the small intestine. This is referred to as the *enteric nervous system*, and like your heart, acts independently of your head brain.

Serotonin, our most popular "feel good" neurotransmitter, is the key player in the gut. In fact, 95 percent of the body's serotonin is used by the gut, not the brain. The enteric nervous system actually contains every neurotransmitter and modulator that is found in the brain. Got your interest? The vagus nerve, a major cranial nerve located in the brain stem, as well as in the wall of the intestines, transmits messages between and the brain and the gut about many things, from function to how things taste.

But for every message sent from the brain to the gut, there are nine sent from the gut to the brain! Good Heavens -- our whole body is a thinking machine!

On the other hand, skeletal muscle also takes some thought, unless it is an involuntary action caused by a reflex in response to a given stimulus. For example, when something flies near your face, you don't stomp your foot; you wave your hand by your face to shoo the object away. Otherwise, external movement takes at least an initial conscious (or unconscious) thought: "I'm hungry." You get up out of your chair and either walk to the fridge and grab a piece of fruit or stuff to make a sandwich, or you jump into your car and drive to the nearest fast food place. Hopefully, you do the first. Either way, you made a conscious decision to move your body.

Luckily for us, we don't have to think about the mechanics of putting one foot in front of the other or opening the refrigerator door; we learned that in *Toddler 101*. But the sequence of movements was orchestrated by a series of nerve signals sent from the brain through the spinal cord nerves to the muscles involved in the motor activity. So, back to the muscles. If you are now convinced that it's better to keep moving than not, you want to learn how to make movement both safe and effective as well as fun. In order to do that, you need to learn *how* that happens. Basically, what skeletal muscles do is to pull bones together or apart. It is the result of muscles in the front of the upper arm that bend the elbow (pulling the bone in the lower arm closer to the bone in the upper arm) and the muscles at the back that straighten the elbow.

Picture this: The bicep muscle group brings your sandwich to your face; the triceps muscles take it away. Not too complicated. During movement, muscles perform one of three tasks. The muscle that actually produces the movement is called an *agonist* or prime mover. The opposing muscle is called the *antagonist*, because its job is to control the speed and force of the prime mover. The third task is helping with the movement. These muscles are called *synergists*.

Obviously, eating a sandwich takes the cooperation and coordination of many, many muscles: the hand, wrist, upper and lower arm (both front and back), along with muscles in the face, head, and neck. It also involves muscles in the chest, side of the ribcage, and the back. (Don't forget cooperation of your good judgment and will power also!) Think how enormous and miraculous that is ... and we never even think about it as we devour that fat, juicy sandwich. The sad fact is we take the miracle of our bodies completely for granted!

Muscles continuously change their tasks -- back and forth, depending on the movement being done. Think of some guys lifting something by a big rope from one place to another, say, cargo from the dock to the ship. One big guy is the head rope puller, and he has a bunch of helpers behind him on the rope. On the dock, another worker is slowing down the pull, and he also has a bunch of helpers. It is the timing, coordination, cooperation, and precision that pulls that off without a mishap. If one person on the pulling end doesn't do his job, the cargo is likely to swing the wrong direction. If his partner on the dock doesn't do his best, the cargo will move too fast, and watch out!

That is the way our body moves effortlessly and efficiently in everyday activities, like taking a shower, getting dressed, eating breakfast, picking up the dishes, etc. So right now let's do another pretend activity. We're going to *Air Swim*. *Air Swimming* is a group of exercises that I originally created as warm up to any exercise class I was going to teach. It provides gentle range of motion in the joints and spiral/diagonal muscle movement for people with chronic pain and for nonambulatory individuals. These exercises can be done standing, sitting, lying in bed or on the floor. They are completely adaptable for almost any physical condition and provide a beneficial effect by increasing blood flow and oxygen to all the tissues of the body, including the brain. They can be done energetically to music or may be done slowly and fluidly as a moving stretch.

Because they cross the midline of the body, they stimulate activity in both hemispheres of the brain simultaneously, increasing signals across the corpus callosum, the white matter comprised of connective sensory and motor axons. This increased activity leads to *whole-brain thinking* and improved focus, concentration, and memory. These movements may be done as a complete group and then repeated several times, committing five minutes or more to the segment. When done this way, the therapeutic effect is *whole body*. They are greatly effective as a mini stretch and brain boost several times during the work day, particularly after hours of driving, desk work, or studying. They are also a great starter for the beginning of each day.

The Swim
Standing or sitting with your legs apart in a balanced position and arms by your side, pull your tummy in and begin a forward swim move. Keep your knees slightly bent. Bending forward from the hips (do not round your back), keep your head and back in line and stroke diagonally across your body in a half-circle. Keep your elbows slightly bent and bring your hand and arm all the way back to your starting position with each stroke. Keep your breathing deep and rhythmic as you swim. Inhaling on the up stroke, exhaling as you come down. Make your stroke big, scooping the air as though you were drawing your arm through the water. Make sure your stroke pattern crosses the midline of your body, ending your stroke at the inside of the same-side knee. Repeat the stroke, alternating arms 12 times. Note: If lying in bed, start with your arms in the Butterfly position. Stroke your arms up, forward and down, bending your elbow as you draw your arm back up to repeat the stroke. (Watch the video for details.)

Back Stroke
Staying in the same starting position as for The Swim, begin to draw your arm up diagonally across you and down to complete the stroke. The back of your hand should be facing you as you start your stroke. Allowing your body to rotate as you stroke, bend your elbows as you bring your arm back and down to complete the stroke, breathing rhythmically as in the first swim move. Keep your tummy pulled in, but keep the rest of your body soft and relaxed as you swim. This is a wonderful moving stretch for the front of the chest and shoulder areas. Move fluidly through the phases of the strokes. Repeat 12 times and follow with the Breast Stroke.

Breast Stroke

Bring your arms forward at chest level, the back of your hands together. Bend forward from the hip, standing up straight as you sweep your arms apart, keeping them extended until they are just behind you. Your palms are facing back. As you reach the back position, bend your elbows and bring the arms back to the front, inhaling as you do that. Exhale on the sweep back, just as you would if you were actually swimming. As you push forward, slightly tuck your chin, allowing the rounding of your upper back. Inhale as you return your arms front, raising your chin slightly to increase the stretch in the front of your body. Repeat 12 times.

Modified Butterfly

Maintain the same wide-legged stance or sitting position, arms at sides with palms facing the side of your body. Raise both arms up over your shoulders, scooping forward and toward the middle. Exhale as you stroke, tucking your chin and letting the thumbs touch before you scoop down, apart and back. The stroke simulates exactly what you would do in the water. As you stroke back, lift your chin and inhale deeply through your nose. Each time you exhale, pull your abdominals in a little deeper, maintaining a stable low back throughout the stroke. Repeat 8 to 12 times.

These swim moves are a fabulous whole body activity that act as both an energizer and moving stretch for stiff joints that have been sitting all day. They incorporate the components of MOPSI: Movement-Oxygenation-Play-Stimulation-Interaction. You can watch the video with someone else to make the movements interactive. Don't discount your imagination here. As I told you before, *play* is big now in science. Part of what can make exercise fun is pretending you're doing something else ... *playing.* Playing you're a flamenco dancer or a matador, or twirling a hula hoop or dancing on the deck of a cruise ship. The more you allow yourself to simulate what you used to love to do (or still do!), the more your brain is engaged. Speaking of pretending, let's work those upper body muscles differently by using a playground ball (about the size of a soccer ball, but smaller and lighter). We're going to be doing a group of exercises using the ball, so get ready to have some fun!

Sitting in your chair or standing, hold the ball between your hands, lift your arms up over your head and bend your arms so the ball is in back of your head. Push those arms back far enough that they don't push your head forward and down. You want to keep your neck relaxed and straight, with your head balanced right on top, as it should be! Doing this to music, of course, increases the fun and the brain's response to the activity … it makes it more fun, of course! Finding the beat to the music (usually a 4/4 beat), lift the ball straight up and lower back down. As you lift over your head, tighten the back of your arms. This is a great activity for tightening those flabby triceps you see when you wave goodbye to someone. Lower the ball back down and repeat the move 8 to 10 times. When this gets easy, increase to 10 to 12 repetitions. You will see results in no time. If you are already strong, you can use a regular soccer ball, but they're heavier and might make you tend to bend your neck forward to clear your head. This is devastating for the neck, so be aware!

Now, to work the opposing muscles, the bicep group: continuing with the ball, hold it in front of you on your legs, palms up, on your knees, with the ball sitting on your hands. Your arms are straight and right next to your ribs. Again, doing the moves to the beat of the music, lift the ball toward your chest by bending the arms in. Then lower back down to starting position on your legs. The palms-up position of the hands automatically causes the bicep group to engage. Do the lift swiftly, then lower slowly. Repeat this 10 to 12 times in a row. Rest and then do another 2 sets of 10 or 12. This may seem like a useless exercise, but believe me, if you sit at a desk all day, or drive a lot, you don't use your biceps much, unless you're a weekend gardener. This won't build big muscles, but the multiple sets will build strength through endurance, an important kind of strength to have as we age.

There are about 602 skeletal muscles in the body, and most of them work in pairs or small teams. As I said, one muscle, or team, pulls a bone one direction, and the *opposing* muscle or muscles help stabilize and control that pull. When the action reverses, the opposing muscle pulls the bone the other direction. They continually change roles. This marvelous bit of muscle and bone movement is called biomechanics. In truth, the body does operate like a beautiful piece of machinery. That's why it is so important to provide it with fuel, water, and rest to enable it to operate efficiently and without breaking down. All movement happens as a result of messages between the body and the brain and from the brain to the body. These messages are carried by nerves. *Sensory* nerves send a message to the brain from some part of the body. *Motor* nerves send the message from the brain to the muscle to move a certain way.

For example: You reach out your hand to pick up a pot off the stove without needing to *think* about how to do it because your brain told your arm to do so. The handle is too hot, so when your hand feels the heat, your arm automatically jerks away because the nerves in your skin tell your brain, "Let Go!" Pretty amazing, isn't it?

Let's go back for a moment to muscle contraction. There are actually two types of contraction. The one that shortens the muscle is called a *concentric* contraction. When this happens, the muscle fibers slide into each other like a telescope. Therefore, a muscle can only shorten to *half its resting length*. The single fibers become double as they slide together. Because they are double strength, they can lift or pull.

Muscle fibers are made up of tissue that is elastic in nature. They can shorten and they can stretch. As a muscle lengthens, the fibers pull apart. If the fibers are still holding tension in them as they lengthen, the fibers experience stress that causes them to break down or tear at a microscopic level. This is called an *eccentric* contraction. Let's do an experiment. Put your hands in front of you, with the palms facing in, your fingers pointed toward each other. Slide your fingers together and squeeze them firmly. This is rather like a muscle that has shortened.

Now, keep that same amount of tension in your fingers and try to pull them apart. Feel the stress? That's what happens inside a muscle if lengthening while retaining tension in the fibers. Why am I telling you all of this? Because I think it is important to know why someone is telling you to do something a specific way. When you understand why, you are much more likely to do it. To build a muscle up, it must experience lengthening contractions that stress it enough to require more protein to make it stronger. The lengthening action *must* be resisted by the person exercising in order to stress the muscle fibers sufficiently. When this happens, the body feels the need to send in more protein molecules either to build up or to rebuild the muscle. This is called *hypertrophy*. It is what causes muscles to become bigger and more defined.

Once again, why am I telling you all this? Because I want you to understand why it is important to lower your weights *slowly* when you are lifting them. By *resisting* the downward or lowering movement during an exercise, you will help your muscles get stronger faster and help prevent injury to your joints. Make sense?

Example: If I tell you to lift the arms only to shoulder level, understanding why can save you a potential injury. Any higher, and you take the move out of the shoulder muscles and into the muscles in the neck. We don't want to do that. The neck is fragile and supports the weight of our head (10% of our body weight) all day long. It's *always* working. The smaller muscles that help support and stabilize the joint that's moving are called synergists, or accessory muscles. Normal, functional movement is synergistic, which helps prevent undue stress to one specific muscle during movement. For instance, when you lift a heavy bag of groceries out of the trunk of your car, you are using many muscles in your legs and hips, your back, and your shoulders, as well as in your arms.

The most appropriate exercises for us older adults are those that use several muscle groups simultaneously, allowing the joints to move through their complete ranges of motion and involving more than one direction.

Think about this. If you are a mother with children still at home, housework can be exhausting, especially after working all day. Unlike many traditional strength exercises that isolate a particular muscle or muscle group, housework uses multiple muscle movements that are involved in normal activities, like doing laundry, lifting groceries, cleaning house, and playing with children or grandchildren. Think about how the rope pulling exercise might make you stronger for raking leaves, or pulling clothes out of a front loading washer or dryer.

If you live in an assisted living situation, where you don't have to do household chores, you still need strength to make your own bed, or pull a coat out of a closet. The practice of pulling movements makes us stronger for even the simplest of activities of daily living. In other words, they make you *functionally* strong. These types of whole body exercises will not only increase overall strength, but will also improve your coordination and sensory awareness, as well as your balance.

We older adults want to include exercises that involve standing on one leg and stepping both backwards and sideways, to familiarize the lower leg muscles with multidirectional movement. When these kinds of movements are not practiced in a safe environment, the brain may not signal the muscles fast enough if you suddenly have to step back up on a curb to avoid being run over, or quickly sidestep a child's toy on the living room floor. These are the situations in which falls occur.

As you learned in Chapter Three, bending and swaying are whole body movements that actually stimulate the vestibular system, particularly the semicircle canals within the inner ear, and ultimately strengthen the nerve networks within the brain. One small sidebar to complete the connection from top to bottom: There is a physical response called the *tendon-guard reflex*, which is a great example of how the brain interacts with the lower legs, feet, and ankles. It is an automatic response to stress -- one of the *fight or flight* responses that dominate so much of our behavior.

For instance, during a shouting match over who got to the lavender sweater (60% off) first, if you are truly riled up at the woman who pushed in front of you and grabbed it, the brain signals the calf muscles to shorten, back of the knees to lock, and your weight to shift (*imperceptibly*) to your toes ... you're ready to stand and fight.

The muscles in the neck and the back contract to keep your trunk stable (if she should shove you!); in other words, you are ready to fight or flee. That *can't* be good for you, but it probably occurs much more than we are aware of in our daily stress-filled lives. Ahhh ... exercise and stretching to the rescue!

So let's take a minute to practice this great lower body stretch that will also strengthen your balance and stability systems. Use the DVD as a training aid, but read through these instructions first so your brain will already have created a picture of what you're going to do.

Tendon Guard Reflex Stretch

Stand facing your kitchen counter or a desk, if it's not too low. Place your right foot flat on the floor, so the toe touches the bottom of the counter or your desk. Next, place your left foot directly in back of your right, as *far back* as you can, keeping your heel down. Steady yourself on the counter by standing so your body is touching it, your hands at both sides. Slightly tuck your chin … not a lot. Don't let the stretch pull your head back up. Now, raise your left heel up and then press it down firmly several times in a row. Make sure your foot is back far enough that you feel the stretch, but you're not holding it down. You're lifting and pressing your heel down about 8 times. This releases the tension in the Achilles tendon and calf muscles and pumps cerebrospinal fluid up and down the spine, including into the cranium, which has three membranes of different thicknesses. The dura mater is the hardest, then the arachnoid, a softer membrane that lies over the crevasses in the brain, and finally the pia mater, which cradles the brain, form fitting to every ridge and groove. This calf pump pushes fresh cerebrospinal fluid through these membranes and the spine, bathing the brain with nourishment that will flow through the body and to all the tissues. As you do this, focus your attention on *feeling* what you're feeling in your legs, in your back, in your neck.

The time it takes to actually stop and notice is microscopic and meaningless within a twenty-four-hour context, or the context of an entire lifetime. But within that stopping and noticing, you have stopped time and acknowledged the miracle of your own body. The flood of wonder and delight at how much there is to notice will probably make you smile. You may even laugh out loud.

You've just discovered *Everything Is Connected* and created your own brain chemicals that support life and boost your immune system. You've also supported your gut brain, which is sending serotonin to your head brain. I bet your heart brain is feeling peaceful. Better than swearing and hitting the steering wheel in rush hour traffic, huh?

■ ■ ■

6

KNOWING THE INS & OUTS

The older adult and senior population has been completely overlooked when it comes to abdominal strengthening. The fact is, we've been abused! Not only are the traditional methods of crunches and curl- ups ineffective and stressful for the younger population, there are actually serious *risks* for the older adult who does them.

What I want to introduce here is a way to think about abdominal strengthening in a whole new light. Not as an uncomfortable, unpleasant, and ineffective method of trying to get the firm, flat tummy you see on the magazine covers (a very unrealistic goal anyway!), but rather as a means of achieving postural stability, a lengthened more youthful appearance, and continuous support for your back and internal organs. This chapter will teach you a method of improving your ability to breathe and a way of toning your abdominal area *while* you also loosen up stiff joints; at the same time, you'll be learning how to give yourself the "core" strength and stability needed to prevent falls.

Seniors and older adults (both men and women) with osteoporosis are in danger of a fracture either to the vertebrae in their neck or in their rib cage from the compression created by curling forward in a traditional sit-up or crunch, even the innocent looking curl-up. This same compression also makes these exercises dangerous for someone with high blood pressure or a history of heart attack or stroke, because of the tendency to hold the breath on the curl-up phase. If you happen to have a lot of abdominal fat, as many older adults do, crunches and curl-ups are particularly difficult to do, and the stress involved in the effort can even put a relatively healthy person at risk for a cardio vascular episode.

Maybe you're one of those individuals who never bothered to do abdominal exercises because you didn't really think much about your posture, and somehow you knew all those crunches wouldn't work anyway. Maybe you're one of the multitude of people who have tried to make yourself do sit-ups or curl-ups every morning, but always hated doing them because they hurt your back. Besides that, they never really made you look any different. Ring any bells? The good news is that there *is* a safe and effective way to strengthen your abdominals. The right exercises can help you stand up straighter, relieve both lower back and neck pain and make you look ten years younger and five pounds lighter. The fact is, they can even reduce your waistline by *at least* an inch and a half! I know you're probably chomping at the bit to find out what these exercises are, but there's still a little more you need to know. Keep reading just a little further.

When the abdominal muscles are weak, there is a bulging of the abdominal wall. Sometimes that looks like the little (or big!) pot belly that hangs over many men's belts, or it can simply be the lack of a waistline that many older women think just comes with age. Even a person with no excess body fat has guts (the internal viscera) that weigh about ten pounds! In either case, there is a downward pull on the abdomen due to the weight of the abdominal contents and gravity. This puts a tremendous strain on the lower back and an unhealthy pressure on the reproductive organs. It also places the diaphragm in a position that affects the ability to breathe and is a common condition in people who are significantly overweight.

The diaphragm is the muscle that opens up the rib cage so the lungs can fill with air. When this important muscle is being compressed due to poor posture and no abdominal support, it can lead to respiratory muscle fatigue and may even precipitate respiratory failure. Lengthening the trunk area -- making room for all the organs to function optimally -- is what happens when you have good tone in the deep abdominals. They lift and support the rib cage, decompress the lower spine, and maintain tone in the pelvic floor. This is a major factor in the health and function of the reproductive organs.

Many of the problems that occur during the aging process may be closely tied to decreased respiratory function. Shallow breathing is one of them. Inactivity, obesity, and the stooped posture of someone with osteoporosis are often involved in the reduced breathing capability that many seniors experience. Poor posture and extended periods of sitting, as well as the metabolic changes that increase the storage of fat around your waistline, all contribute to the overstretched abdominal wall we observe in so many older adults. (Look in the mirror lately?) To make matters worse, these overstretched abdominal muscles play a predominant role in the weakened postural muscles in the back, increased compression in the hip sockets, lower back, knees, and feet, and reduced circulation to the legs.

Finally, these weak muscles affect the functioning of the intestines, bladder, kidneys, and prostate, because the organs are not supported sufficiently within the abdominal cavity.

Are you finally convinced? Let's try a couple of the exercises that can get you in touch with these deep muscles, then I'll tell you a little more about them. Let's begin by teaching you how to breathe.

Belly Breathing

Lie on your back with a rolled towel or pillow under your knees, or sit comfortably in a straight back chair. Lengthen your spine. If you are lying down, extend your arms out in a diagonal, up from the shoulders and relax the back of your hands on the floor. If you are seated, let your hands relax in your lap. Close your eyes and *feel* your body weight making contact with the surface you are on. Keep your back lengthened, but relaxed, and relax your abdomen. Now, inhale deeply through your nose and pull the air all the way down into your midsection. As you inhale, *feel* your belly stretch and move outward. As you exhale, *feel* your belly gently move inward.

Important note: If your chest rises up first and your belly pulls in as you inhale, you are reverse breathing (or chest breathing). Keep practicing until you feel the difference. The tendency is trying too hard to relax and consequently over breathe or hyperventilate.

Okay, let's take this a little further and actually begin to *work* those abdominal muscles! This next exercise lets you *use your muscles to pull in as you exhale*. The key is to exhale slowly and forcefully through pursed lips, like you were blowing out a candle. This allows you to control your breath and really feel the muscles pulling in. Think about pulling your abdomen *all the way back to your spine* while you're exhaling. When you need a new breath, just relax, breathe in deeply through your nose, and let your tummy stretch.

Active Belly Breathing
Begin to lengthen and slow down both your inhalation and your exhalation. Breathe comfortably through your nose and keep your chest and shoulders relaxed. As you breathe in slowly, allow a greater stretch in the belly. As you exhale slowly, begin to *actively pull in* throughout the exhalation. Don't force the length of your breath. Allow your body to establish its own rhythm.

As you feel yourself getting more relaxed and breathing easily through your nose, intensify the pulling in *on the exhale*. Imagine a string on the inside of your belly button, and pull it all the way back to your spine. Continue this for a few minutes, envisioning the deep abdominal corset wrapping around your body and *feeling* the elasticity in the muscle fibers. Hold the muscles in deeply until you feel fatigue and need to release. When you relax your contraction, do it slowly to retain the muscle memory in the deep abdominals.

Do this about four times, resting in between -- but do not do more. More is not better. More *often* is. Although the concept of trunk stability (the center of your body) may be somewhat new to you, the idea of a connection between good posture and good health is probably not. I bet your mother always told you to "stand up straight!" The idea of a correctly aligned body in relation to feeling good (and looking good) has recently made a comeback in many health and wellness magazines; and currently the importance of balance and postural stability for seniors has been getting a lot of attention. The problem has been that they are still selling traditional abdominal exercises to address this issue. This simply doesn't work!

"Trunk stabilization" refers to stabilizing the center of your body by strengthening the muscles that hold the rib cage and the pelvis in correct alignment. This is important because when these two large bony parts of the body are not aligned properly, the weight distribution on the spine is uneven, and all the joints in the body are affected. When the trunk is unstable, and the core muscles are weak, the risks for falling are greatly increased because the body doesn't have the strength to correct itself when it starts to tip!

Yet, even the very elderly and frail have a need for trunk stabilization. Those individuals who are completely dependent on someone else's care also need to have core strength and stability to avoid injury when they are being moved from bed to wheelchair, or even turned. Needless to say, the caregivers must have core strength to avoid injury when moving someone's body. Very often, the elder person is so frail they are basically dead weight.

Traditional approaches to abdominal strengthening can't be used. Seniors with problems getting down and up off the floor are also omitted. Seniors with respiratory problems can't do them. Seniors with osteoporosis or cervical spine problems and DDD or DJD (degenerative disc disease or degenerative joint disease) certainly should not do them.

Anyone with a history of high blood pressure, heart attack, or stroke are at risk because of the compression on the main arteries when curling up, and those with a lot of abdominal fat find it almost impossible to lift their upper body up. Here is a gentle, feel-good method of gaining true abdominal strength. If you can get down on the floor, or lie down on your bed (provided it's firm!), that's great – but even if you can't, you can do this sitting in a chair. This is the first level of adding resistance to those abdominal muscles.

Because you are going to hold your tummy in this time and go back to regular breathing, your breath actually puts "resistance" against the abdominal muscles from the inside! This will make them stronger much faster. The key is to keep the rest of your body relaxed while you breathe and hold your tummy in. It's difficult as first, but trust me, you will learn how. Soon, it will come naturally.

Basic In and Up

Inhale deeply through your nose, allowing your abdomen to expand. Exhale through pursed lips, forcing most, but not all, of the air out, and pull your abdominals *in and up*. If you are lying down, you may feel a slight rotation of your pelvis move your lower back toward the floor. <u>Don't press your back onto the floor.</u> If you are seated, don't drop your chest as you exhale. Keep a lengthened spine. Hold that position the best you can, with your buttocks relaxed. Go back to breathing easily through your nose. Don't let your tummy expand when you breathe in. Keep holding it in.

Hold your abdominals *in and up* deeply, feeling your tummy sink in and up under your ribs. Count to ten as you continue to breathe, and pull in a little deeper on your abdominals. Imagine a string attached to the inside of your belly button. Pull that string in toward your backbone and up under your ribs. *Keep breathing.* At the end of your count of ten, relax and return to deep belly breathing. Repeat 2 or 3 times. How do you feel?

The Breathworks program that I created in 1989 and published as a book in 1998, *BreathWorks For Your Back Strengthening Your Back From the Inside Out,* is where these exercises come from. The BreathWorks program focuses on the deepest layers of your abdominal muscles, to create a firm, internal corset of support for the center of your body and lower back.

The exercises involve no bending forward or curling up and can be done in virtually every body position. This gives you a means of attaining core strength and stability no matter where you are and even working for those confined to a bed or wheelchair.

With the newly learned (or often relearned) concept of pulling the abdominals "In & Up" you can achieve strengthening of the deepest abdominal muscles, improve your posture, and experience easier, fuller breathing through the daily practice of belly breathing. These gentle exercises also provide a way of attaining a deep state of relaxation and assisting you when things are stressful.

This is the way it works -- your abdominal muscles are the primary muscles involved when you exhale. When you breathe in, the diaphragm expands and moves downward into the abdominal cavity to allow air to be drawn into the lower lungs. As your diaphragm expands, the small muscles in between the ribs lift and stabilize the rib cage as the lungs fill, and the air reaches the upper pockets of the lungs. The breath is exhaled in reverse, first leaving the upper chest, down through the rib cage, and lastly is *pushed* from the lower lungs by an inward movement of your deep abdominal muscles.

The stronger the deeper abdominal muscles are, the greater their ability to compress the abdomen and push the air out when you exhale. This is very important for anyone suffering from emphysema because the inability to fully empty the lungs is one of the difficulties in their breathing. You can go to my website: nancyswayzee.com and see examples of what I'm telling you.

Although I am rushing you somewhat, I want to teach you a second way to add even more resistance to these muscles. This next exercise not only strengthens your abdominals, it also strengthens and stretches all the muscles in the upper back and shoulders. Because you do this lying on your back, this exercise can also be done by someone confined to a bed. If you need to do it seated, simply position your arms as directed. It will work the shoulders more because your arms are not being supported by a flat surface.

Important: Only move in a range that is comfortable for your shoulders. Full range of motion is not necessary, nor desirable, if you have a history of shoulder problems or surgery. This exercise will create and maintain muscle strength and support for the shoulder joints and alleviate the stiffness that comes from being immobile.

Angels in the Snow -- Alternate Arm Move

Lying on your back, with a pillow under your knees, stretch your arms out to each side, with the palm facing up. Your arms should rest on the floor at about shoulder level so that your body forms a "T." The back of your hands are on the floor.

After doing some Belly Breathing, inhale, and let your tummy stretch. Then exhale and pull your abdominals in deeply. Now hold them in and go back to breathing easily through your nose. Keep your tummy in! Begin to move your arms slowly like a windmill, sliding one arm up next to your head as you slide the other one down next to your hip. Keep the palms facing up and your tummy pulled in. Do this slowly, 5 or 6 times.

On your last repetition, leave your arms in the windmill positions – one up by your head, one down by your hip. The arm by the hip, turn the palm down. Moving them at the same time, begin to slowly sweep them up and down in a straight line. Bring one arm down as you bring the other arm up. Take the arm sweeping up as far as you can comfortably. Do not move into pain … *listen to your body*. If you have full range of motion, allow the back of the hand, on the arm up by your head, to touch the floor. Immediately continue on with your series of sweeps. Keep your arms straight, and repeat this 5 or 6 times. Do it slowly, and keep your tummy pulled in and breathe easily. Last, let your arms meet at the center of your chest, and open back out into your "T" position, with the palms facing out.

Keeping your arm straight as long as you can, bring your right arm across your body (chest level), touch your left arm and return to the floor. Now repeat with your left arm … bringing it over to your right. Do this slowly 5 or 6 times, keeping your abdomen pulled in tightly and breathing easily. Next, slowly lower your arms to your sides. Relax your body and slowly release your abdominal muscles. Go back to deep, belly breathing. What do you think about that? Pretty tough, huh?

This next exercise is basically the same set of moves, but done standing or sitting. Standing is preferable, if you are able. This dramatically changes both the impact and the intensity of the exercise. When you are on your feet, the weight of your internal organs, as well as the gravitational pull, adds significant resistance to those abdominal muscles.

Being upright also makes the exercise more functional, because it is teaching your body to support its weight (and your back) while you are doing your everyday activities. This is very important! If you are able, do this in front of a mirror so you can make sure you are keeping the top of your shoulders relaxed.

Standing Alternate Arm Move

Stand with your feet hip-width apart, arms at your side. Relax your shoulders and think about lengthening your spine. Inhale deeply and allow your midsection to expand. Exhale through your mouth and pull your abdominals in and up.

Notice your rib cage in the mirror. Your goal is to hold the center of your body very still as you move your arms. Holding your tummy in firmly, raise your arms to chest height, your palms facing forward. Begin to move your arms *slowly* like a windmill, keeping your palms facing front. Slowly move your left arm up toward your head as you bring your right arm down next to your hip.

Keep the movement going, reversing and going the opposite direction. Keep your tummy in and up! If your shoulder movement is restricted or stiff, only go up as far as you can go without discomfort. Keep repeating this movement for about 6 times, trying to move your arms at the same pace ... and remember – slowly!

While keeping your tummy in, leave one arm up by your head, with the other by your hip, palm facing back, and begin to sweep your arms over the front of your body, just as you did on the floor. Keep the top of your shoulders relaxed and don't let your back arch as your arm moves over your head.

This will feel very difficult, especially since you are holding your abdominals in tightly and breathing! Repeat this about 6 times, slowly return your arms to chest height and then relax them by your side. Good job! This is pretty intense neuromuscular reeducation. Doing this every morning before you get dressed (so you can see your tummy) will result in strong abdominals, a firmer, flatter tummy and much better posture!

This chapter is an important one for you because knowing how to support the center of your body makes it safer for you to do everything you do as well as the strengthening exercises and the fancy footwork.

Practice these exercises every morning and every night. Do one or two repetitions of each one (no more). During each repetition hold your tummy in until you feel your muscles getting tired. If you are faithful about these exercises, you should begin to feel and see a difference in about two weeks. Good Luck!

■ ■ ■

7

TAKIN' IT ON THE ROAD ... PORTABLE EXERCISES

This chapter is all about portable exercises. In other words, exercise you can do anytime, anywhere. They require no specific equipment, no amount of space, no specific clothes. Nothing is required except your strong intention and attention. Yes, that's what I said -- attention. The fact is, I'm teaching a class right now called "Exercises for Anywhere." As word has spread, the class has gotten very popular. The students are from their 60s to late 80s. The key is, of course, that all the exercises are adaptable to every age. They can be made more difficult, and they can be made easier. The class is tailored to fit the individual students.

The idea is that these are exercises that can be done in an RV and/or in an office cubicle. Some of them can be done while riding in a car, or even in an airplane. They are small, unobtrusive, and very, very effective. They are great for long road trips. You just step outside the car and do the ones for the lower body -- very good for stiff legs and hips and sore backs after hours in the car. These are also good for taking a break from sitting at a computer hour after hour.

The most appropriate exercises for us older adults are those that use several muscle groups simultaneously, allowing the joints to move through their complete ranges of motion and involving more than one direction.

Exercises that use multiple muscles reproduce the physical movements involved in normal activities, like doing laundry and housework, carrying groceries, working in the yard, and playing with grandchildren.

They make you *functionally* strong. These types of whole body exercises will not only increase overall strength, but will improve your coordination and kinesthetic awareness as well as your balance. In the last chapter, you learned about strengthening the abdominals. It is equally as important to strengthen the other postural muscles: the muscles in the back and of the butt (gluteal muscles).

To familiarize the lower leg muscles with multidirectional movement, I include exercises that have you standing on one leg as well as stepping both backwards and sideways. These movements must be practiced in a safe environment. The brain may not signal your muscles in time when you must quickly step back up on a curb of a busy street, or quickly sidestep a child's toy on the floor. These are the situations in which a fall can occur.

Bending and swaying movements actually stimulate the vestibular system, particularly the semicircle canals within the inner ear, and strengthen the nerve networks within the brain. These movements, as well as coordinated movements of the body, "wake up" the neocortex of the brain where we do all our thinking. That's a great reason all on its own!

Here's a fascinating side note: The Center for New Discoveries in Learning found that music with 60 beats per minute, such as might be found in Mozart's music (which activates the left and right hemispheres simultaneously), increases learning and retention of material by up to five times. In addition, this beat pattern "resulted in a recall rate by almost 100 percent, even after not reviewing the material for several years." Now, you probably won't be doing these exercises to Mozart, but standard pop is 120 beats per minute, simply two sets of 60. The only music that doesn't work is hard rock. The brain actually shuts down and can go into a state of anger or subconscious thinking when hearing too many repetitions of a line. Believe it or not, the muscles in the body actually go weak. Put on some mellow Frank Sinatra, Stevie Wonder, or Paul Simon, and let's get ready to learn. We will talk a lot more about the importance of music and rhythm in the next chapter.

Our focus is to attain and maintain strength, trunk stability, balance, flexibility, endurance, coordination, agility, and reflex response; to insure our ability to live vital, healthy lives and be able to perform the activities of daily living, self-care, and recreation with ease and energy.

One of the ways we do this is to exaggerate the functional moves . . . make them bigger and slower or smaller and faster, or some combination of both. We add resistance in whatever form is appropriate for you, the reader/student. Naturally, some situations may require a slightly different approach. Let's say you are already a fairly fit individual, but now you have a particular fitness goal you want to achieve. Perhaps you've decided to run your first 10k race, or enter in a triathlon for seniors. CONGRATULATIONS!

Maybe you already run, but now you want to take a bicycle tour around the country, or are planning to hike up Mt. Whitney. Possibly, you already have great endurance. Now you want to actually *build* some larger muscles. What if you are currently living a healthy lifestyle, have a lot of energy, and have a regular exercise routine that is keeping you fit and maintaining your weight, but you've noticed you are much stiffer in the morning than you used to be; or maybe it's just getting harder to get up after you've been sitting a long time, or working in the garden is harder to do because getting up and down from the ground is more difficult. If that is the case, then these exercises are also good for you.

If you have severe arthritis (as I do), getting down on your knees can be really uncomfortable. The best way to prepare yourself for these exercises, if you feel stiff, is to precede them with the Going Around in Circles or Swim Move exercises. Both of these provide a total body warm up for the muscles and joints and will make any exercise much more comfortable.

If you are planning for a *specific* type of activity or have a particular problem you want to tackle, then your training would also be more specific. Regardless of the particular thing you want to prepare yourself for, you have to begin by getting *basically* fit.

These portable exercises are actually great for targeting specific muscle groups for strength, but done in a manner that replicates something you might do every day. For instance, getting up and down out of a chair (or the toilet) is an activity we need to retain all of our lives in order to retain our self-sufficiency and our dignity.

Most kitchen and dining room chairs as well as sofas and overstuffed chairs are between 17 and 18 inches high. A regular toilet (not handi-capped) is under 16 inches. That's actually pretty low and requires at least a 90 degree knee bend in most adults. I'm only five-one and have very strong legs. Yet my arthritic knees speak when I have to lower myself down. Thankfully, my thighs are strong enough to always lift me back up. Unfortunately, that is not true for many, many seniors. Approximately 90 percent of falls in the elderly take place in the bathroom.

All the portable lower body exercises that follow help to build and maintain bone and muscle strength, flexibility, and balance … all neces-sary in the execution of lowering down to sit and lifting the weight of your body back to a standing position. So, let's get right to a couple of easy ones.

Sit to Stand

Sit toward the front of a flat-bottomed chair that is approximately 18 inch-es high. If you need to place a flat pillow on the seat to make it that height, do so. Your back is lengthened and your feet are about hip-width apart. Keep your arms close to your body with your palms resting on the front of your legs. Pulling your abdominals in and up to support your back, inhale deeply through your nose and push down through the bottom of your feet, raising yourself to a standing position. Raise your arms to chest level. *Slowly* lower down and back as though sitting on the chair. As you lower your body, keep your arms at chest level. This will help give you bal-ance. Lower your body until the back of your thighs *lightly* touch the chair, returning your hands to your knees. Then, push back up to a full standing position by pushing down through the bottom of your feet. *Do not allow your body weight to sit on the bench.* As you stand back up, squeeze the muscles in your fanny. Inhale as you sit back, exhale as you stand up. Continue the squat move for 2 sets of 4 to 6 repetitions, focusing on using your breath to assist you. On the last repetition, lower your body weight down even slower and immediately begin the next exercise. As you get stronger, you will increase your repetitions to sets of 8.

The key here is to squeeze both cheeks tightly when you're standing up and really stick your fanny out in back when you're sitting down. That's total flexion and extension, or simply put, shortening and lengthening of the gluteus maximus muscle. Do this every other day. For best results, don't let your fanny rest on the chair. Simply touch and immediately stand back up. Let's say you aren't quite strong enough to do the Sit to Stand enough times in a row to make your muscles stronger. You have to start *smaller*, with Body Bouncing. Yep, another totally silly exercise that has incredible results! This one will really tone your thigh muscles.

Body Bouncing

Stay seated with your legs hip-width apart. Your feet are directly under your knees, at a 90 degree angle. Put your hands on your thighs so that your fingers are touching both the outside and inside of your legs (check the DVD to see the position). You're going to be gently squeezing your legs as you do this in order to *feel* how strongly the muscles are working. Once again, when you do this to upbeat music, it's twice as much fun.

Sitting up straight, with your tummy pulled in, simply press down through the bottom of both feet, as though you were going to stand up. *Slightly* lift your bottom off the chair … but not quite. As soon as you press down, you release, so you sort of "bounce" your bottom on the chair. You're going to do this to music again, to have a rhythm to bounce to. Every time you press down with your feet you are going to feel all the muscles in your legs get tight. After you have done this 6 to 8 times, you are going to start to feel fatigue in your thighs. This is a major strength move that most people never even think of! When you can do this for 10 to 12 times, you're on your way.

Let's keep on moving … down. Now to the fanny itself, and everything from the bottom of the ribcage down. This next exercise doesn't need much description of what it does. You'll feel it.

Seated Gluteal Squeezes

Sitting on your flat-bottomed chair or bench, place your feet flat on the floor, with your knees at a 90 degree angle. Lengthen your spine, relax your shoulders, and pull your abdomen in and up. Squeeze your cheeks together firmly, and hold for a count of 4. Repeat this 8 times (remember to breathe). Now do a series of 8 fast, tight squeezes, and hold the squeeze on the 8th squeeze for a count of 4. Repeat this routine 4 times, keeping your tummy pulled in and up the whole time. While you are holding the squeeze, envision the abdominal cavity as a box -- a top, four sides, and a bottom. *Make the box smaller.*

Pull *everything* in and up. For women, the cervical muscles are circular, so screw them down tight, as though you are tightening the lid on a jar. Squeeze as though you are trying to stop the flow of urine.

Men -- you do the same thing. Squeeze and lift everything inside. This is a great way to strengthen your entire abdominal wall, as well as the muscles in your buttocks. It's important to breathe comfortably throughout the exercise. The tendency is to hold your breath while you're holding the squeeze. Your fanny will feel tired afterward, and you may even have some sore muscles the next day, but that's just a sign you worked these large muscles well!

I'll let you in on a little secret -- these squeezes have a great benefit for both women and men. I'll tell you the secret by sharing a letter I included in my first book, *Breathworks For Your Back Strengthening Your Back From The Inside Out.* Here it is:

"After fourteen years of marriage, your abdominal and pelvic exercises have certainly brought a new level of excitement into our lives." The letter was from the wife. The husband took his wife and me out to a wonderful dinner!

Just this last week, a student in her 80s came up to me after class and whispered in my ear, "My husband says this class is making life better for both of us." As I walked out to the parking lot, she and her husband drove by and he gave me a "thumbs up."

Although you may see dozens of other more complicated exercises for a firm fanny in the glossy magazines at the grocery checkout line, these two exercises are all you really need to do. They strengthen the muscle "functionally" -- meaning they make the muscle strong practicing what it needs to do in real life. These two exercises can give both men and women great, firm behinds!

Let's keep on going. You want to be able to stand upright after you've been sitting for a long time, rather than remain hunched over and shuffle. Unfortunately, there's not a lot that can be done about the stiffness that comes from arthritic changes in the bones. That is simply a result of wear and tear on the body and is usually more severe if you're overweight or have a history of joint injuries. I bet you notice the stiffness is worse when you *haven't* been moving! Like first thing in the morning, when you get out of bed, or when you've been sitting for a long time.

I've got some great moves to ease that stiffness, but they come later in the chapter. Getting back to the lower body, let's talk a little more about the butt, fanny, or bottom (to be clinically correct, the gluteus maximus). This is the largest muscle in the body, and together with whatever body fat you have, it makes up the curve or shape of your buttocks. A firm, rounded mound of flesh is what makes a baby's butt so adorable.

The gluteus maximus muscle is attached on the back and side of the thighs, just under the cheeks. During hip extension, the fibers contract inward and upward, pulling the leg backwards. The weight must be off the foot for this to happen. Although its primary function is hip extension, this muscle also has a prominent role in standing up from a sitting position -- and in standing back up after squatting down. Next time you have the chance to observe a toddler, watch them squat down to examine things and then stand back up. They may do this continuously all day.

The muscles in the front of the thigh are what straighten their legs and lift their body weight from the squat, but it is the contraction of the muscle fibers in the back and the buttocks that return their little body to an upright position. Here's why: As the toddler stands up, the gluteus maximus muscle contracts the *opposite* direction from extension, and pulls the buttocks down toward the back of the leg, stabilizing the stance. Pretty complicated sounding, I know, but actually elegant in the simplicity of the mechanics. Everything works together at once ... smoothly. This is the miracle of the body.

That toddler's little teetering motion when first coming erect is a combination of muscles that have not yet developed full strength; undeveloped muscle memory, and the vestibular system telling the brain to use the muscle in their legs and feet to assist in gaining balance. Wow!

In retrospect, this is what happens to any frail individual who has been bedridden or incapacitated for a long time. It has very little to do with aging -- its lack of muscle use! Unfortunately, a shapeless, sagging hind end is what you usually see on older adults, both men and women. Believe it or not, you can do something about that.

There are plain facts we need to get out of the way. First of all, a small waist makes a fanny look shapelier, and the cold, hard truth is that we do get thicker around our middle as we age, both men and women. Even if we don't have excess body fat, we tend to store what we do have, right around the center of our bodies. This is just nature's way. Although you do occasionally see them, an hourglass figure is pretty rare on someone over 50. The abdominal exercises you just learned will GIVE you that waist back. If you do the In & Up exercise every day, that's a guarantee.

There's another thing that contributes to a fanny that *appears* less shapely. As we age, many of us lose our lumbar curve due to decreasing disc size. This decrease in the discs may be caused by degenerative disc disease, specific disc injury, or just years of compression and dehydration.   In any case, the result is a flat-back syndrome. When the normal low-back curve that we had as children and younger adults was there, the rear end is accentuated and can look shapely even when there is very little muscle tone. When there is no lumbar curve, the shape of even a *fabulous* fanny is less evident. Nevertheless, you can have a firm fanny.

The shape of your butt is usually determined by genetics, but if your activity is ice-skating or ballet, you're likely to have a pretty well-developed backside regardless of your family's body type.

The two exercises we did before focused more on the flexion phase of movement than on extension. Although the Sit to Stand does have extension in the standing phase, it is more of a leg strengthener than a butt exercise. Because the *primary* function of the gluteus maximus is hip extension (moving or lifting your leg behind you), the activities that incorporate that position will develop and maintain this large muscle. This includes standing up from a sitting or squatting position.

Lifting and holding your leg out in back like a skater or a dancer creates a well-developed, shapely muscle. You can recreate this move without ever putting on a pair of ice skates or ballet slippers. (You may want to view the DVD on this next one, to make sure your form is correct.) Sometimes I call this "The Skater's Butt" exercise.

Standing Back Leg Lift

Stand, holding on to the back of your chair. The back of the chair should be about waist high. Lengthen your spine and open your chest area, so you feel taller. Now, pull your tummy in firmly, put your right leg in back of you, with the toe just touching the floor. Turn your toe out slightly. Make sure you keep your left knee soft; don't lock it back. Squeeze your right cheek tightly. Just for fun, reach back with your right hand and *literally* squeeze your bum … feel that? That's muscle, my dears. Hold your leg up for a count of 4, contracting your cheek tightly, and then lower slowly. Repeat this 10 times.

The key here is to keep your tummy pulled in deeply. If you don't, you're likely to arch your back and create uncomfortable tension in your lower back. If you have a hard time feeling this, place your hand firmly on your abdomen as you lift. If you want to know a more advanced way of doing this, rest your body on your dining room table with your feet still on the floor, or even your bed (if it's firm), with your feet on the floor. Keep your knees slightly bent. Lift your right leg out behind you (making *sure* you are pulling your tummy in), and straighten it out as much as possible, squeezing your butt. Hold for a count of 4, and repeat this 10 times.

Then change to the other leg. Your goal is to have your leg level with your back. This is not easy, because the body wants to twist. Do your best to keep your back level. You should be able to *feel* this, but if you can't, practice with someone else and have them put a 12 inch ruler right across your low back. Try to lift without letting the ruler slide off. That's level!

Doing this in a horizontal position makes it more advanced because you are holding your leg up against gravity. If you want better results, try turning your toe out slightly. The gluteus maximus muscle also rotates the leg, so lifting your leg with a slight external rotation of the foot will make the muscle stronger faster. **Just don't overdo**.

After you have completed this, place your foot on the seat of the chair and rest your chest on your bent leg. (Make sure you *steady* yourself!) This allows your lower back and butt to stretch out. Hold this for a count of 10. Repeat this with the other leg. If you want the best results, do this 2 times a day, every other day. Not every day, because this is a large muscle, and needs to rest in between strengthening sessions. Don't forget to stretch it out afterwards, or you will experience even more delayed onset muscle soreness than you ordinarily would. If you're faithful, you should begin to see and feel increased firmness and tone in about a month. Wouldn't that be fun?

A muscle gets strong specific to the move it is trained to do ... and you need to be able to do other things besides get up and down out of a chair. One of the most important components of leg strength is how strong they are individually; *kneeling* down places one leg in front of the other, not side by side. The leg in front is bent at a 90 degree angle from both the hip and the knee, with the foot flat on the floor. The leg in back is at a comfortable distance in back of the front thigh, with the ball of the back foot on the floor. Both knees need to be able to bend to lower you down, and both legs need to be able to lift you back up. Kneeling also requires balance so that you don't topple over. Balance is one of those functions that lessens with age, and there is some physiological basis for that change. Make sure you steady yourself with a chair-back or counter top, even if you think you're balanced enough to do it without.

The center for balance is the vestibular system, located in the inner ear. This is the first system to develop in utero. The vestibular system controls our sense of equilibrium and balance, mainly in the head and directly relative to gravity. It is monitoring our positioning during movement and when we are holding still. The inner ear is a group of small organs and canals and vestibular nerve cells that are sensitive to the changes in the endolymph fluid as it flows over the tiny hair cells within the canals. When the fluid moves, the tiny cilia bend, sending a message to the brain about where our head is. As we right ourselves, and the fluid moves, the hair cells return to their upright position.

One of the major changes that occurs as we age is a decrease in our ability to rehydrate our tissues. Over a lifetime of use and oxidation, our tissues dry out. This doesn't affect just our skin, which is exposed to the elements -- it affects all the tissues in the body. It's one of the reasons the discs in our spine become thinner and more brittle, and the synovial fluid in our joints loses some of its viscosity, resulting in less cushioning between our vertebrae and in the joint capsules. Even our eyes dry out as we get older.

Not only can the same thing happens to the endolymph fluid in the inner ear, making it become thicker and flow less smoothly over the tiny hair cells, but lack of sufficient physical activity causes those vestibular nerve cells to deteriorate and cease to function.

The result is poor balance and a decreased kinesthetic sense of "where we are in space," making a person much more vulnerable to falling. By the way, did you know that 20 percent of people who sustain a hip fracture die within a year? Probably the most serious loss is that of attention. When you can't or don't hear what's going on around you, you quit paying attention. As I said before, attention is crucial to learning and retaining information. A lot of what appears like short-term memory loss is that the person simply didn't notice what was going on or was said.

But the news isn't all bad. *That's* only one of the systems that deteriorates without physical activity. All the systems and tissues in the body require blood flow, carrying life-sustaining oxygen to function.

Those vestibular nerve cells die because of lack of their essential nourishment. Get moving, and those cells don't have to die of starvation. Okay, I'll get off my soapbox. Obviously, there are other factors that can cause unsteadiness or dizziness and increase the risk of falling, but lack of leg strength doesn't have to be one of them! So let's get back to kneeling.

The following is a simple, safe way for you to practice kneeling, strengthen the muscles in your legs, and gain more confidence in your balance. Remember to get permission from your health care provider before doing any of these exercises.

You can do this either holding onto the backs of two tall chairs, or a chair and some other piece of furniture. If you have pretty good balance, but want a terrific way to strengthen and tone your legs, you can do this just lightly touching a banister or countertop for support. If your balance is good, do it free - standing. You will get an even better workout, because you'll be using additional muscles that come into play maintaining that balance. One secret of maintaining balance, is to focus your eyes on a spot somewhere in from of you, that is eye level. Keep your eyes focused on that spot while you are practicing your balance.

Stationary Lunge

Holding onto your chair or counter if you need to, place your right leg directly in front of your left leg, as wide as you can comfortably go. Raise up onto your back toes. Now stand up straight and hold your tummy in and up. Bend both knees and slowly lower yourself down about 2 inches. If you're just beginning to exercise, keep it a small bend. If you are usually pretty active, this could be several inches, but not more than 4 or 5 inches at the most. Your back heel *stays lifted* and you are going to feel a stretch in your back leg. Keep your body right in the center of your legs -- don't lean forward as you're lowering *straight* down.

Using the chair or counter for balance only, push through both your feet and raise back up to a standing position and squeeze your back cheek tightly. Stay up on your toes on your back foot. If you feel some stress in your knees, don't lower down quite so far. *Otherwise,* you want to be able to keep mobility in those joints, so don't be afraid to try. If you were able to do this successfully, repeat that move 8 times. Inhale as you lower, exhale as you straighten your legs and squeeze the cheek of the back leg. If you're just not able to do it 8 times, do it as many times as you can -- even just 4x will eventually make you stronger. Because the front leg and the back leg are working the same muscles a little differently, it's important to work both sides ... repeat with the left leg forward.

Get your legs apart, stand up tall, tummy in, and lift your back heel. Remember, use your chairs only for balance. You want to make those legs stronger, not put the stress on your shoulders and arms.

Important: You don't want to do this if it causes you actual pain, particularly in the knee or hip joints. This exercise is difficult and does require a certain amount of strength even to do one. Feeling discomfort in the muscles in your legs is to be expected, but pain is not, and should be paid attention to!

If your knees are hurting, make the knee bend much smaller, and make sure you're not leaning your body forward. This will transfer your body weight onto your knees. If your hip joints are hurting, try adjusting the width of your legs. Either take them a little further apart, or bring them a little closer together. Keeping your abdomen pulled in deeply is crucial. If you don't, you are likely to arch, and this will bother your lower back.

There's a lot to remember, isn't there? That's okay, it is truly worth the effort, and you can always use the DVD to help you maintain good form. Think how much easier gardening will be when kneeling down and getting up is not such an impossible chore. Spontaneous weed pulling is just like picking a piece of lint up off the floor. You don't usually stop to think about it. You don't get out your kneeling pad or stool and position yourself for a lengthy bout in the garden. You see a dandelion or a dead flower, and boom ... before you know it you've gone down on one knee to correct the situation. THEN you try to get back up! Sound familiar?

Let me tell you about all the muscles you were using when you were doing this simple exercise. First of all, you're using all the deep and intermediate muscles in the back and neck to support your head and trunk when you are upright. You're using all the abdominal muscles to align and support your rib cage in relationship to your pelvis. They keep your rib cage from tipping forward, which would round your back, and they keep it from tipping backward, which would arch it. They play a very important role in maintaining your balance while you are doing this exercise.

You're obviously using the gluteus maximus (the butt) because one leg is doing hip extension (the leg in back) all throughout this exercise. If you really squeeze your cheek on the back leg as you push back up, that will aid in developing that nice, rounded, firm behind.

You know you're using your thigh muscles because you can *feel* them. They are probably talking pretty loudly right now … saying, "Holy cow! What are you doing to me?" By the way, the Oil Derrick exercise in Chapter Three is another great way to retrieve something off the floor, and it's also a portable exercise! Remember to stabilize yourself with a piece of furniture or a countertop if your balance is at all shaky. By the way, all of these exercises are a version of bending over to pick your shoe or sock off the floor, so they are *totally* functional.

In clinical studies done on groups of older adults, one group exercising, the control group not, results have consistently shown a reduction in falls up to as much as 46 percent in those who exercised regularly. One of the very best forms of exercise for balance is Tai Chi. Tai Chi is an ancient dance-like form of movement that focuses on shifting the weight from one leg to another in a variety of positions. Because the arms are moving simultaneously in slow, graceful sweeping motions, many muscles come into play, assisting the body to maintain balance. In one of the largest studies done, the adults that practiced the Tai Chi moves reduced their risk of falling by 40 percent.

A lot of unsteadiness occurs because the ankles are wobbly. This is often referred to as "canoe legs." Pretty accurate description, isn't it? Well strengthening the muscles in the lower legs can help this. The next exercise not only works the calf muscles but helps keep good circulation in the lower legs and feet. The key here is to stretch well afterward to avoid sore muscles and leg cramping. Instructions for stretching correctly are at the back of the book. Stepping off a curb and crossing the street is always a challenge. If your ankles are wobbly, watch out! This is a time when falls can occur: all your body weight is suddenly on one knee of one leg. This is a place where knees and ankles often fail.

Standing Single-Leg Knee Bend

Once again, holding onto the back of a chair for support, lengthen your spine and pull your abdomen in and up. Lift your left foot and tuck it behind your right calf, so you are just standing on your right leg. Soften your right knee, don't lock it back. Keep your weight on the back half of your foot, directly under your ankle. Bend your right knee, lowering your body down about 3 inches. If this causes pain or discomfort, only lower 2 inches to begin with. By pressing up through your heel and ankle, straighten your leg and return to your starting position. Now, lift your heel and go up onto the ball of your foot. *Slowly* lower back down. Repeat this move 8 times if you can. Repeat with the other leg.

The key here is not to lean forward at all and to keep your body weight directly over your ankle. This will keep your weight from being transferred to your knee. It may help your balance to keep your buttocks contracted while you do this.

This is a great exercise for both strength and balance. As you progress, try holding on to the chair with one hand. Coming up on the toes is often the biggest challenge for your balance. As with any of the exercises in this book, do as many as you can. Don't be intimidated by my suggesting 8 to start. If you can only do 4, start there. It's only the beginning. The thing to remember is that all of this has to do with preserving the highest quality of life ... for the rest of your life. In order to be able to continue to do all the things we love to do now -- and want to do in the future -- we need to maintain health and strength, and avoid accidents and injury the best we can. That means *actively* participating in self-care.

One of the best "self-care" activities is walking. If your daily activity is normally sitting at a desk or driving, get up or park and get out, and walk around your area 3 or 4 times every couple of hours. Walk energetically, swinging your arms and breathing deeply. The people around you may think you're a nut, but what do you care ... you'll be a healthy nut and have a much better attitude than they do -- take my word for it!

Actually, about 12 or 15 years ago, when I was teaching for Tahoe Forest Hospital, they arranged for me to go to the local PG&E office, where most of the employees sat at a computer all day. I taught them all of these portable exercises that could be done at their cubicle, doing the stairs and walking the halls, when they had their 15 minute breaks and on their lunch time. They loved it. They would come back to their desk so energized, their performance increased dramatically!

We only have now. So it pays to notice. Here's another great portable exercise that will allow you to *feel* the process of muscle contraction. This exercise is for the back of the arms, the triceps; but it also works the muscles in the chest, shoulders and upper back. Remember, the job of muscles is to pull bones toward and away from each other. The particular job of the triceps muscle is to straighten (extend) the elbow. The muscle is attached at the back of the shoulder blade and at the top of the forearm at the back. The muscle contracts towards the back of the shoulder and pulls the lower arm away from the upper arm. Now that you have the picture, stand in front of your kitchen counter, or a piece of furniture that is "fixed" so it won't move with your body weight. If you're in a motel or hotel, use the bathroom counter or the writing desk that's in every room.

Triceps Press Up

Place your feet about 18 to 24 inches away from the counter, and place your hands on the edge, with the fingers pointed more or less towards the center. (Use the DVD for reference.) Let your shoulders relax. *Do not hold them up towards your ears!*

Keeping your heels on the floor, bend from the ankle and let your body down towards the counter. Keep your tummy pulled in and your back in a straight line. Your body wants to move as a unit. Bend from the ankles and not the hip or you'll be throwing the exercise away! As you *slowly* lower down, your elbows will bend. Keep them pointing out to the sides and let your chest touch the counter edge. Keep your legs straight (knees soft) and heels on the floor. Push back up to your starting position by *slowly* straightening your arms. (Feel that?) Repeat as many times as you can to fatigue. Rest, and then do another set to fatigue.

This is a great exercise for the upper body and you can do it anywhere, even at your desk at work. As you lower down, in addition to feeling the stretch and strain on the back of the arms, you should *feel* a good stretch in the chest. You will also *feel* the muscles between your shoulder blades pulling them together and the stretch between them as you push off. Lots of stuff to feel ... great opportunity to get to know your body.

It's also a great way to tone the back of your arms. How does this relate to survival? Well, if you were to take a fall, your triceps need to be strong enough to raise your upper body off the floor so you can push up onto your hands and knees to begin the process of getting back up. If you were in any kind of an accident where you were trapped between or underneath something, the ability to push the object away could save your life. Dramatic? Yes, but factual. A simpler example, how about pushing a heavy box where you want it to go, or pushing a heavy drawer closed? How about trying to close an overstuffed suitcase? That is everyday life. Do you still get down on your knees to say your prayers? This is how you push yourself back up. Simple!

A little bit of muscle trivia . . . the triceps rotate the palm *down*, the biceps (next muscle we're getting to), rotates the palm *up*. So let's do one more exercise for the back of the arm -- and you'll be doing this, but you may not think about what you're doing with your hand until you look *up* at it! Yes, I said up. Here goes:

Triceps Overhead Press

Standing with your feet hip-width apart, with a can or weight in each hand, bend your elbows and rest them on each shoulder. (Look at the DVD.) The ends of the cans or weights are facing front and back, your palms are facing down toward the shoulders. Press your right hand up over your head, straightening your elbow and *rotate your palm forward*. Tighten the back of your upper arm firmly. You will feel the muscle contract. Return the hand and arm to starting position and repeat with the other arm. Do alternate arms for a series of 10 to 12 repetitions.

Now, do one more and look at the position of your hand as you rotate ... the palm is facing forward, or down if your arm was straight out in front of you. Amazing isn't it? The position of the hand totally determines the muscle group you are working! Good job. Okay, let's move on.

Now we're going to look at the front of our arms, the biceps. One more bit of muscle trivia here: The reason the triceps sound plural is that although it is only one muscle, it has three heads, or separate parts, that all work together to produce the end result. Oh, and that rotation thing. Well, the muscle doesn't do the rotation on its own; the three heads work as a group with several other muscles to accomplish the turning over of your hand. It's the same thing with the biceps: this large muscle has two distinct parts, attached at slightly different locations (as is true of the triceps) and works together to *smoothly* perform flexion or bending of the elbow.

Every time you pick up your coffee mug, it's your biceps that do it. When you set it back down on the table, it's your triceps at work. But remember, these two different muscles are working together during both actions, otherwise you'd splash coffee all over your face and smash your cup when you set it back down. The body is a miracle of synergism ... everything coordinated and working together to make life possible, efficient, and lasting for as long as we take care of it!

To make a muscle stronger, you have to stress it ... yes, I said stress it. Because homeostasis works on a negative feedback system, things won't get bigger, stronger, faster, or looser until the particular body system has been asked to do something difficult or impossible. Remember, **Use creates demand, demand creates function;** same formula as the brain thing. When you ask the muscle to lift something heavy and you don't have the strength, the protocells in the muscle will send out its message, "More protein. More protein. I need bigger fibers." So, the body responds and gets to work building more fibers and more capillaries to allow more blood flow, enabling the muscle to accomplish the task.

The standard formula has been that when you discovered what amount of weight you could lift once, but no more, then you took between 70/90 % of that amount and lifted it to fatigue (so you can lift it practically forever and not get tired). When you can lift something about 8 times before fatigue, you up the amount of weight and start over.

What actually happens when you first start is that lifting the weight causes microscopic lesions in the muscle fibers (called micro-trauma) from lifting the loads. Delayed Onset Muscle Soreness is caused by micro-trauma, not lactic acid, as we once believed. Two things happen: The body builds more muscle cells and the cells get bigger. Which one happens, and which happens first is dependent on who's doing the strength training and how hard they are doing it. The muscle actually increasing in size is called hypertrophy.

This is a highly simplified way of describing what actually happens, but the effect of the lifting is stress and so the body jumps in to help reduce the stress by giving you more muscle. I once had an instructor in a physical therapy course say, "Exercise is simply controlled injury." He was right, and I regularly tell my classes, "Remember, weights are WMDs (weapons of mass destruction), so handle with care!"

On to the exercise. Many magazines and other programs suggest using filled gallon milk jugs as weights for the biceps. I personally disagree. Holding that much weight *below* the wrist puts an incredible strain on the joint. The handle is also uncomfortable for arthritic hands. Using something that will have the weight in line with the hand is the safest way to lift. Chances are, if you are reading this book, you are just starting out. Let's either use the kidney bean can idea (approximately 1 lb.), vinegar or olive oil bottles (about 2 lbs.), or what the heck, wine bottles (a little over 3 lbs. ea.).

When you're ready to get serious, buy yourself some 3 lb. and 5 lb. weights and go for it. Until then, improvise. Remember, these are portable exercises, so use what's handy.

Biceps Curl

Stand, or sit, in flat-bottomed chair with feet flat on the floor, knees shoulder-width apart. Holding your cans, water bottles or 2 or 3 lb. weights in each hand, hold your arms (palms up) all the way out to your knees. Your weights are resting in your palms. Bend your arms, lifting the weights up all the way to your shoulders. *Slowly* lower back down to starting position. Inhale on the lift, exhale on the lower. Use a slow count of 4 on both the lift and the lower. Repeat 8 to 10 times. Do 4 sets of repetitions. Simple exercise. Let's make it a little more energetic. Same exercise, but done as a series of fast pumps. The key is absolute control of your movements. So, here we go.

Biceps Curl Pumps

Stand with your feet hip-width apart, holding weights at waist level. If seated, sit on the front of your chair, with feet flat on the floor, directly under your knees. Weights are still resting on your knees, elbows touching the ribcage with your palms facing up. Lengthen your spine and pull your abdominals in. Relax your shoulders and breathe.

Begin your pumping curls, alternating your arms, from the waist position to the front of the shoulder. Make the moves fast, crisp and controlled, maintaining tension in the muscles. Do not relax between the lifting and the lowering phases. Repeat this pumping action for two sets of 12 and rest. (Refer to the DVD if you aren't sure.) If you feel energized and want to try, do one last set of 12.

You have just begun the process of sculpting beautiful, toned arms. I don't care how old you are or how wrinkled your skin is. Muscle will help to fill in those sagging arms. Congratulations!

Two very important things to pay attention to when you are strengthening the front of the arm: do not over extend (straighten) your elbow. When you get to the bottom of the lowering phase, your elbows still want to be soft. That's an exact description of how it should look, a very small, soft bend. Second, you want to work *within the frame of the body*. That's why you're resting the back of your hands on your knees.

Keeping your lower arms in line with your upper arms protects the elbow joint (as does keeping the soft bend) and the inside of your upper arms next to your ribcage. Now, you can hit the road with confidence. Your vacation doesn't have to mean abandoning your fitness routine. You are taking it with you!

■ ■ ■

8

BACK TO A KID AGAIN . . .
PLAY BALL!

I am going to have a ball just writing this chapter. It was about ten years ago that I discovered the versatility and value of a playground ball when teaching exercise. It began when I created my Breathworks for Your Brain class. I saw it as a safe, usable tool to create and improvise both individual and partner exercises. Bouncing or tossing a ball, whether playground or tennis ball, demand concentration, rhythm, coordination, reflex/reaction. This activity uses both large and small muscles, eyes and ears, and the vestibular system (balance/inner ear). The primary brain areas involved are the basal ganglia and the cerebellum, both responsible for motor control and organization of our thought processes.

Dysfunction of the basal ganglia is involved in Parkinson's and Huntington's diseases. Within the basal ganglia lies an area called the substantia nigra, which produces dopamine. Dopamine is an important neurotransmitter for sending and receiving signals between neurons in the brain that control movement. When the production of dopamine ceases, movement becomes involuntary. This results in the tremors involved in Parkinson's disease and the jerky movements in Huntington's.

One of my first activities with the Parkinson's patients I work with is replacing involuntary movement with voluntary movement, i.e., bouncing or tossing a ball. It works! This has been my approach to Parkinson's from the beginning: *Replace involuntary movement with voluntary movement.* This has proven to be effective every time.

The problems: It takes motivation and consistency, something that many Parkinson's patients don't have. It only works while it's being done. It is not a cure, but it does seem to slow down the progression of the disease. Because there are so many different individual phases and stages, each person's response to the voluntary movement approach is different. Human beings -- all living beings, whether plant or animal -- are not textbook. That's why none of us can know the absolute and conclusive answer to problems, or even some questions. What we *don't* know will always be greater than what we do know.

But back to playing ball . . . Once again, music is an integral part of the activity, because rhythm is a necessary component to the body and the brain. Rhythmic movements are what stimulate brain development in an infant. Babies naturally begin to rock back and forth on their backs, instinctively developing the strength to roll over to their hands and knees. These first natural rhythmic movements open the door to sensory awareness and begin to connect the parts of the brain. They create and develop balance and tactile awareness (what they feel on their skin, with their fingers, and with their hands). The sensation we feel when we move our muscles is called *proprioception.*

These three components of information have access directly to the neo-cortex and affect the ability to focus, to control impulses and emotions, and to learn skills such as planning, abstract thinking, and creativity. This early rhythmic movement also plays a part in the development of language skills, information processing, retention, and memory. This is why every activity in this book is linked to music and rhythm, and using these two components when playing with a ball is also FUN!

In my exercise classes, we use playground balls for at least half of the class. Something as simple as stepping side to side, while bouncing a ball, takes great concentration and focus. If the beat of the music is fairly fast, you can't take your eyes off of the ball, or you'll miss it when it comes back up to you.

To avoid a stiff neck from just looking down at the ball, we alternate bouncing and tossing and catching. Each person has their own ball. My students are all different sizes, i.e., I'm five foot-one, another woman is about five foot eight. From outside looking in, it looks a little like a circus act. Everyone is doing their own type of step, everyone is laughing, even hoopin' and hollerin'. Everyone leaves the class energized and in a better mood than they were when they came in. When doing this activity, you are totally "in the moment." Problems disappear, worries are forgotten.

When we shift to partner activities with both balls, it gets really crazy. We all partner up. I try my best to put people who are close to the same size together, but sometimes that is difficult if the class is small. Nevertheless, we stand about 3 or 4 feet apart, facing each other. The instructions are to simultaneously bounce the ball to your partner's left foot. This means that you are bouncing from your right side and catching on your left . . . shifting quickly, and repeating it . . . over and over again. This activity involves so many senses and systems at one time, it is incredibly challenging; but everyone is laughing and having so much fun, our immune systems are all shouting, "Yeah!" and getting stronger by the minute. Laughter is one of the strongest immune boosters there is.

This fun game requires using eyes, ears, hands, arms, and feet in co-ordinated movements to the rhythm of whatever music is playing. This is a true *whole-body/brain* activity, while producing major BDNFs at the same time.

We repeat the same thing, only tossing to each other, rather than bouncing. Tossing to each other is more complex than bouncing, because the concentration must be continuous; identifying and focusing on the area of your partner's body you want the ball to go for easy retrieval by them. The toss must be simultaneous, or it throws the rhythm off, and keeping a volley going is impossible. Very, very complex, and an enormous amount of fun and GREAT for the brain!

When we are going for a more cardio-intensive workout, we hold the ball against our chest, arms tucked into sides. Then, we alternate pushing the ball out and back in, and pushing it up and then down. As we push forward, we say "Out -- In." As we push up over our heads, we say,

"Up -- Down." We do this to the beat of music (of course), and I urge them to speak loudly to use their lungs and vocal chords. Even the 80 year olds in the class can do it. Everyone works at their own pace. It is a GREAT exercise. We are all breathing hard and smiling when we're done.

For a more cerebral activity, we stand in place and say our times tables out loud as we bounce the ball. Of course, it's rhythmic. We repeat the 2-4-6-8s out loud to 100, and do them all up and through the 9s. It's a great retrieval game, and all of us are challenged with our 6s, 7s, and 8s. Additionally, to challenge our concentration, I divide the class into two groups, and have one half bounce and sing "Row, Row, Row Your Boat," while the other group bounces and sings "Twinkle, Twinkle, Little Star." This is another one that gets us all laughing. My advice: Get a playground ball (the cheap ones are fine) for you and anyone else in your household, go out on the patio, the deck, or even your kitchen floor, and PLAY BALL! Once you start, you'll never want to stop.

I Guarantee it.

■ ■ ■

9

SSTTRREETTCCHHING . . . . .
THE TRUTH

This chapter is very important because the exercises are not strenuous. Nevertheless, they work and tone the large muscle groups effectively. When muscles have been contracting, they need to return to their resting length by the process of stretching.

Every muscle in the body is attached at an oblique angle. This oblique orientation is what allows spiral/diagonal movement. Herman Kabat, MD, PhD, the noted neurophysiologist, first developed the PNF modality in the 1940s and, recognizing the spiral/diagonal nature of it, created therapeutic exercises with diagonal patterns to develop strength *and* flexibility.

When a muscle is stretched diagonally, the muscle tissue is affected all the way to the end of the musculotendinous junction, where the tendon attaches to the bone. The cumulative effect of muscle elongation that occurs as the movement is continued allows enough time that the Golgi Tendon Organs (GTOs) release their inhibitory response and allow the muscle to stretch. The GTOs are one of those sensory receptors I wrote about earlier that register a "too much" of anything condition and take their appropriate action. The GTOs initially stop a muscle from stretching until it is sure it isn't going to be pulled off the bone; that takes about 20 to 30 seconds. Then the GTOs send the signal to the muscle that it can relax and stretch. The longer you hold the stretch, breathing throughout the stretch and moving the body part gently to increase the stretch, the better stretch you will get.

For many years, we were told to stretch before beginning to exercise. Now we understand that static (held) stretching of cold muscles results in damage to the muscle tissue and can cause injury. We have replaced pre-exertion stretching with warming up. A good warm-up prevents muscle strains and tears by gradually increasing the flow of blood, oxygen, and fluids through muscle tissues. The good news is all these stretches can be done in a working environment. Simply find a chair that is as flat as possible. A bucket chair won't do. These stretches may also be done standing, if you have good balance and can find surfaces that are the right height. *My suggestion would be to watch the DVD and do the stretches along with it when you are first starting. Stretching is necessary and good for the muscles, but, if done incorrectly, can cause injury.*

The most efficient way to stretch is from the bottom up, because when standing or walking, the foot is at a right angle to the ankle and calf. When we roll through our foot as we walk, tension is carried from the bottom of the foot, through the legs, into the pelvis, gluteal and back muscles, all the way up to the base of the skull. Therefore, we start by stretching the bottom of the foot, the ankle, and the calf. Then, we move to the back of the thigh, the hamstrings, the buttocks, the sides of the body (which stretch each half of the back muscles). Then, we move around to the hip flexors, the front of the thigh, the front of the lower leg (the shin area), and the top of the foot.

Next, you stretch the side of the body by doing a stretch that affects the back of the arms (the triceps), the small muscles between the ribs, one half of the back, and even reaches down to the outside of your hip. Next are the biceps and the chest muscles (one side at a time), and last, the middle of the back, all the way down to the pelvis and including the sacral area (the bottom of the pelvis). Finally, you stretch the neck. By this time your muscles have all let go of their tension, and you should feel light as a feather and fully relaxed.

I've led you through this road map before explaining the actual stretches in order for you to see as well as feel the logic in stretching this way. One important note: This full body stretching is only necessary after a complete exercise class, workout, bike ride, or power walk. When doing only the small exercises in this book, specific stretching of the body parts involved is all that's necessary. You may do this full body stretch after cleaning house, working in the garden, or any other full body activity.

To start: Stretch the calf, the ankle, and the bottom of the foot. Use an area that is anywhere from 4" to 6" high, like a curb, a step, stair, or a low hearth. If you don't have access to anything like that, you can use any vertical surface: a door jam, the leg of a chair, or the corner of a wall.

Stand facing the surface, about 2 feet away. Obviously, your height will determine all these distances. Standing on your left foot, with the knee soft (not locked), put the ball of your right foot and toes against the surface. Your heel is on the floor. The right knee is straight, but also soft. Standing tall, back lengthened, chest lifted, tummy pulled in, take a breath in through your nose, and as you exhale through pursed lips, bring your chest forward towards the surface you're facing. Bending from the ankle, your body stays straight. You will feel the stretch first in the ankle and the calf. As you continue to press your chest forward, you will feel the stretch in the bottom of the foot and behind the knee. When you have reached the point of discomfort (not pain!!!), hold that position, breathing easily through your nose, and count slowly to twenty. At that point, gently rotate your toe inward. You'll feel an increased stretch in the outside of your right lower leg. Hold and breathe for a count of 8, then slowly rotate your toe outward, the stretch moving slightly to the inside of your calf. Hold for 8, breathing easily, then return your foot to center as you return your body to your starting position. Repeat the entire process with your left leg.

Next, moving to the hamstrings in the back of the leg: Because of balance issues with older adults, doing this stretch sitting is the safest and most effective way. Sitting on a flat-bottomed chair, like a kitchen chair, sit close to the front, with one foot on the floor, directly under your knee. Extend the other leg out, with the heel on the floor, toe pointing up. Place the same side hand on your knee, other hand on top of it. Take a deep breath in through your nose, and as you exhale through your mouth, slide your hands down your leg as far as you can go. You're bending from the hip, not the back (very important!). Keep your chin tucked, do not let your head pull back. Hold quietly, and breathe as you count to twenty slowly. You can gently rotate your foot both inward and outward as you stretch. On completion, place your hands on your knees and push yourself back upright. Do not use your back. Repeat with the other leg.

Now, for the front of the thigh, the quadriceps, four very large, powerful muscles: Usually, they are very tight, as are the hamstrings, so be patient. As you do these stretches daily, you will find the muscles lengthening and stretching with less resistance. You need two surfaces to do this stretch. One you can hold on to, to steady yourself, and one the right height to place the top of your foot on. If you have had surgery of the hip, leg, foot, or ankle, consult with your doctor before doing this stretch. The flat-bottomed chair you used before is great to stabilize yourself with. You can use either another flat-bottomed chair, or if just starting out, a small, flat-topped kitchen step stool works great.

Stand facing the surface that you are stabilizing with, i.e., the back of one of the chairs. The surface you are using to stretch on needs to be in back of you, at a distance where, when you place the top of your foot on it, your thighs are together and the bent knee is pointing straight down. Bend your knee on the leg you are stretching and place the top of your foot on the surface, with the bent knee leg fully supported. Keep your knee soft on the standing leg. Pull your tummy in, lift your chest, and lengthen your back. Squeeze your buttocks tightly, and gently press your pelvis forward. Holding on to your chair for support, lean your upper body back, just until you feel the stretch in the front of your thigh. Hold for a slow count of twenty, breathing throughout your stretch. When done, carefully remove your foot and place it on the floor. Repeat with the other leg.

Moving to the upper body: Stand with your feet about hip-width apart, tummy pulled in, back long. Place your left hand on the side of your left leg and lift your right arm up next to your right ear. Bend your right elbow and allow your arm to rest on your head. Inhale deeply through your nose, and exhale through your mouth as you bend to the left, sliding your left hand down your leg. Go as far as is comfortable and hold. Feel the stretch down the back of your right arm, all down the side of your body, and even into the top of your right hip. To return to standing position, place your left hand on your hip, and press yourself upright. Do not use your back to straighten up. Repeat with the other side.

Next, the front of the arm (the biceps), and one side of your chest: Standing next to a doorway, raise your right arm to about chest height. Curl your fingers (palm down) around corner of the door jam, on inside of door. Holding firmly, inhale deeply through your nose, and as you exhale through your mouth, rotate your body around to the left, creating the stretch in the right arm, shoulder, and chest. Relax the top of your shoulder and breathe easily, counting to twenty. Repeat with the other side.

Now, to stretch the back: Stand with your legs hip-width apart, tummy pulled in, back lengthened. Make a circle with your arms, directly in front of your chest, fingers interlaced. Relax the top of your shoulders. Soften your knees, gently round your back, put your head face down, in the circle, and carefully move the circle to the left as far as you can comfortably go. Stretch forward with both arms, really pushing out with the back of the right forearm. Feel the stretch in the entire right side of your back. Hold and breathe, increasing your stretch by pushing out with your right arm. Gently move the circle to the right, and repeat. Return to center, take your legs wider apart; put your hands on your knees, then do a small rotation with your fanny. Tuck your pelvis under -- stick your fanny out in back. Repeat this pelvic rotation 4x, then push on your knees back up to a standing position.

Last stretch: The neck. Cross your arms in front of your chest, hands on your upper arms. Let your arms drop and rest on your chest. Notice which arm is on the outside. Tuck your chin to your chest and gently roll as far to the right as is comfortable. Keeping your chin down, gently roll to the left. Repeat the rolls 2x. Return to center, raise your chin to level, and turn your head as far to the right as is comfortable. Look over your right shoulder with your eyes. Slowly return to center and repeat to the left. Return to center and repeat again. Returning to center, re-cross arms with the opposite arm on outside. Repeat entire neck stretch series. When you have finished, return to center and rest, taking in a few deep breaths through your nose, exhaling through your mouth. You have just stretched your entire body. Feel pretty good? I know you do. I do this at the end of every exercise class, and my students LOVE IT!

■ ■ ■

10

FINISHING UP: SURVIVAL OF THE FITTEST

This miracle of our body is simply mind-blowing. We exist because the instinct to survive is hardwired -- stay alive at all cost, and for one reason, to propagate our species. Every species of everything wants to be the biggest and the best and make as many duplicates of themselves as they can; even our cells have this native intelligence.

In *The Feeling of What Happens,* Antonio Damasio, one of the worlds most respected neuroscientists, states,

"We begin as a nonconscious grouping of cells, which beget the neural signaling that creates the proto-self. This new organism establishes a base out of which our core consciousness arises and our core self is born. As the neural pathways develop our sensory system, allowing us a means of taking in information and experience, our autobiographical self begins to build which will lead us to the pathway of extended consciousness."

So, let's talk about the proto-self for a moment. According to Damasio, the proto-self is constantly constructing and reconstructing a map of the state of the body at all times. Yet, even though these cells are theoretically nonconscious, the fact is they communicate with one another, checking in all the time to see if "everybody's okay." This method of communication is called signal transduction. It is part of the process of homeostasis. It is the language of life. Damasio says that when *any* change or sensation is registered by our sensory system, it immediately signals the proto-self to make the necessary adjustments to maintain homeostasis. The signals are neuro-transmitters: brain chemicals scurrying back and forth in the form of molecules.

They exchange the molecules (like those message carriers that tear around San Francisco on their bikes). The hand over is a type of electrical charge, called a synapse . . . the transfer of the message of life.

Interestingly, we operate very much like an ant colony. The body is the queen ant, the molecules are the workers. It *all* comes back to chemistry and electricity, the stuff that created the universe. Hmmm, lots of big words here. Bear with me. Homeostasis is easy. Remember? We talked about that earlier. It simply means a balanced state of being. Everything functioning the way it's supposed to. When the proto-self picks up the news that something is slightly out of whack, let's see ... you just had a re-ally close call by another driver who almost ran you off the road. You pull over, you're breathing hard, and your heart is pounding.

Our breath is tied directly to our emotions, as are all our body systems. Fear, anxiety, anger, agitation all result in a flood of brain chemicals and hormones that speed up the aging process by causing cellular breakdown and death. Rapid heart rate, increased blood pressure, rapid, shallow chest breathing; all these things occur as blood is shunted away from the other organs and fingers and toes and go to the large muscles preparing them for fight or flight. The release of adrenaline causes the body to break into a sweat and, because digestion stops, we may feel nauseated. Dr. Ira Glick, a professor of psychiatry at Stanford, said: "Behind every emotion and piece of behavior, there is a change in a molecule."

The same kind of relay goes on when you enter a walk-in cooler at the deli, to pick up the five-lb. block of cheese for the party. Your body gets goosebumps and you start to shiver. That's the proto-self telling your thalamus to tell the little muscles under your skin to start contract-ing and relaxing really fast to create some heat. You get the idea. All of this happens without our ever noticing – but that's the point. If you notice -- I mean really pay attention -- you might actually *feel* the process. Every part of your body is equipped with receptors(we talked about this before), that tell your brain what the state of your body is; and all of this is for the purpose of survival. We've spent our lives taking this all for granted. We abuse ourselves without even thinking: "It's ok, a few more hours of work won't kill me." "What do you mean, don't shout? I'm really upset!" "Give me a pack of Marlboro Lights, will you?" or "That's all right (lifting a big box), I can get it."

Before we go any further, stop and notice if anything hurts. Just be perfectly still for a moment and feel. As I'm writing this, I'm standing, and both my feet hurt and so does my low back. My body's telling me I need to take a break. What about you? Does everything feel hunky dory? Is your neck stiff from looking down at this book? Put it down. Get up and roll your shoulders, walk into the other room. If you're reading in bed, put the book down for a moment and take in a few deep breaths . . . with your eyes closed so you can feel the breath entering your nostrils. Then slowly release your breath through your mouth. Take a minute and stop time.

That is all the exercise we're going to talk about in this book. Let's get back to *Play*. Paying is what children do -- movement is what children do, because they do it for *fun!* Young children are aware of their physical bodies. Very small scratches, imperceptible splinters, and tiny bruises are investigated daily for changes. Band-Aids and soothing ointments become terribly important to assuage the insult to their little bodies. They express great concern for their mortality, and want to share the news of their "boo-boos" with almost anyone who will listen.

With the exception of acknowledgment when they're tired, most children are tuned in to their body's needs. They eat when they're hungry, won't when they're not. They usually know when they're too warm or cold, and they say when something is too tight. They speak up if they can't see or hear something. They want to touch things with their hands or mouths in order to send the sensory information to their brains. From the beginning, they explore their bodies, fingers to mouths, hands to hands, fingers to toes, hands to genitals. Without the ability to understand or use words, their experience in the world is based solely on their ability to *sense* things. Their sense of sight, sound, smell, taste, and touch. They are completely physical.

On the other hand, we adults go to church to get close to God. We go on a hike to get close to nature. We go to the gym to get fit. We go to the company picnic to get close to our boss and co-workers. We go to Thanksgiving dinner to get close to our family. We go to weddings, baby showers, and cocktail parties to get close to our friends. We stay completely removed from *ourselves*. Our proto-cells are screaming at us to slow down and take a breath and/or a drink of water . . . or maybe a walk in the park, woods, meadow, wherever would nourish your soul. Do we hear the cry for help? Usually not.

One of my fellow authors in *Audacious Aging* is Bruce Lipton, PhD, who is also author of *The Biology of Belief*. He is a cellular biologist who did pioneering research on cellular life (stem cells, in particular) at Stanford University. In *Audacious Aging*, Dr. Lipton describes how life began as single-cell organisms that learned how to split themselves apart to produce progeny because community life was easier than single life. Two can live as cheaply as one!

At that early stage, cells didn't die, they simply split into pieces and kept on going. The problem began when they started to split so many times that they began to fragment. Their "splitting" mechanism wore out. They just couldn't split themselves up anymore. Cells began to "age" and die. Sounds like what I was just describing, doesn't it?

In *Wherever You Go, There You Are*, Jon Kabat-Zinn says, "We fall into a robot-like way of seeing and thinking and doing. In those moments, we break contact with what is deepest in ourselves and affords us perhaps our greatest opportunities for creativity, learning and growing. If we are not careful, those clouded moments can stretch out and become most of our lives."

Back to Bruce Lipton . . . He writes: "Neuroscientists have found that the conscious mind controls our biology less than five percent. Ninety-five percent of our behavior and our choices are controlled by our subconscious mind. The subconscious directs what are called stimulus-response programs, i.e., habits. Habits free the conscious mind from having to pay attention."

Here's some good news. A recent article in *Scientific American Brain* -- "Where Mind and Body Meet" -- wrote about what I'm talking about here, noticing the sensations in your body. It turns out that people who are tuned into their body are more adept at tuning in to other people. Surprised? Not me.

At the Institute for Cognitive Science, in London, several research tests on different groups of people were run. The objective was to determine if a connection between what is called emotional intelligence (the ability to correctly read your own emotions) and the ability to *feel* the physical sensations produced by your body could be found. The tests consisted of matching a sound beep to their heartbeat, without any stethoscope or other monitor. The brain scans showed a lot of activity in several regions, but in those that could accurately feel their own heart, there was increased activity in something called the "frontal insula." Yep, you guessed it. It's in the neocortex that lets us *think* out our emotional reactions.

Have you heard the expression, "Use your grey matter"? Well, the test group that could feel their own bodies the best had more grey matter, i.e., more *thinking* brain. It was actually thicker! I'm telling you, it pays to notice.

So, how do you develop this skill if you have been just leasing space in your own body and you don't even *know* the landlord? You simply start now. It's never too late. Your body's been waiting for you to come home. One of the best ways to do that is with exercise. Let's change that to *Active Physical Movement*. APM creates so many sensations in the body because of increased blood flow: warmer muscles, increased body heat, etc. So here's one last upper body exercise (also portable), that will give you a great opportunity to *feel* all those physical responses!

Punching Bag Boxing

Stand facing an imaginary opponent, with feet shoulder-width apart, back lengthened and abdominals pulled in. With your arms at mid-chest level, palm down, punch using alternate arms. Keep your elbows lifted, wrists locked and elbow slightly bent at point of contact. Pull fist back at the same speed as you throw it out. Do not snap elbow. Allow the punch to move diagonally across body at chest level. Do not try to make this a fast move. Concentrate on rhythmic smoothness of the move. Keep the top of your shoulders relaxed. Use a steady count of One, Two. I have my students say, *"Push / Pull."* Involving the language centers of the brain just intensifies the body's motor response. Repeat 10 to 12 times. Do two sets. Wasn't that exhilarating? That kind of energetic activity is the best RX for depression, hopelessness, fear of aging, lack of confidence or just the blahs.

You know what? You ARE fabulous! Man or woman, fifty-something or eighty-plus. You are ready for this. You are willing (You're reading this book, aren't you?) . . . and you're obviously able. I take my hat off to you! We can't undo or change the past, and the future is only time that isn't here yet. Now is the only thing that's real. Now is all there is ... You can do this. NOW!

Sooo -- This is where we say goodbye. I've given you everything I have to give on this fascinating subject . . . our miraculous, magnificent housing while we're here on earth, our physical body, and its necessary partner and roommate, our brain. Because they cohabitate, they must get along, and in order to get along, they must communicate. I sincerely hope you have enjoyed this book. I hope, too, that you have gleaned some wisdom regarding the need to pay attention to what your body and brain are telling you about the care and respect they deserve.

Nancylister Swayzee

POSTSCRIPT

Finishing this book has been my best experience of "self-actualization," and completely exhausting. The title has changed three times, from Breathworks for *Your Brain* to *Wholebody/Brain Breathworks*. It sat since 2010 in its varying stages while I created and taught Breathworks for Your Brain classes, had open heart surgery, and did some acting and cabaret singing. In between those events, I went back to a novel I had started in 1984, wrote two children's books, and began writing music with a talented composer. All this *bizziness* kept me from following my own advice or practicing what I preached in *Moment by Moment ... An Ageless Process*, which I published in 2011. Here is a paragraph from the chapter "Paying Attention":

"Yet, with all our good intentions, we still get sidetracked. When we stop paying attention, things, people, activities, obligations, etc. begin to overfill our lives. It's like the Peter Principle of the purse . . . the bigger the purse, the more stuff you put in. You keep upsizing the purse, but it's futile . . . the bigger the purse, the more stuff you "stuff" in. When we do this, and we won't listen to our heart, our body steps in and begins to sends its own signals. Irregular heartbeats, midnight anxiety attacks, low back or neck pain, headaches, chronic stomach and bowel problems. Remember *dis-ease* does lead to disease.

In May of 1993, a year of many tragic events in my life, I was still trying to recover financially from my second divorce and move from Colorado back to California. I was working three jobs and was trying to get my private practice off the ground. I wrote in my journal: *I became aware of these new physical symptoms back in October, when I took the train from Colorado. The symptoms were severe pain in my hands and my hips, and the old ones -- my low back, my feet -- returned. My back and feet hurt each time my fear about money surfaces. I wonder, how do you really integrate a new belief? How do you apply it when the numbers are evident and the obligations are looming? I do believe that everything will be provided for, but my body still responds to my not being paid yet and the rent is due and I'm behind in my loan payment. My body is in constant pain, but how can I stop?*

But I did. At least I slowed down, and thank God, I was continuing to journal, so I was keeping in touch with myself. Like everyone else, I found (find) it harder to walk the walk than to talk the talk. My life has been a series of falling down and getting back up. So finishing this book is about paying attention (once again). This time it's about noticing/paying attention to the connection between our body and our brain, how miraculously they communicate with one another and with us. When we don't pay attention to the signals they are sending, we pay the price -- in both physical and mental health well- being. I sincerely hope this book makes a difference in your life. Writing it has in mine.

nls

BIBLIOGRAPHY

Smart Moves - Why Learning is Not All in Your Head 2nd Edition- Great River Books 2005 Carla Hannaford, Ph.D.

Train Your Mind, Change Your Brain - Ballantine Books 2008 - Sharon Begley

Spark- The Revolutionary New Science of Exercise and the Brain -Little, Brown & Co John J. Rately, MD with Eric Hagerman 2008

Brain - The Complete Mind- How it Works, and How to Keep it Sharp - 2009 Michael S. Sweeney, Foreword by Richard Restak, MD

Neuroscience - Second Edition- Sinauer Associates, Inc. Publishers 2001 Stanford University Text

Textbook of Medical Physiology, Seventh Edition - A.C. Guyton, MD

BIOMARKERS - The 10 keys to Prolonged Vitality - William Evans, Ph.D and Irwin H. Rosenberg. MD - Simon & Shuster 1991

Play - How it Shapes the Brain, Opens the Imagination, and Invigorates the Soul Penguin Group New York Stuart Brown, MD with Christopher Vaughn 2009

Dance and the Brain - University of CA, Santa Barbara - The Dana Foundation 2009 Grafton, MD, Cross, MS

The Serious Need for Play - Scientific American Mind 2009 - Werner

Auditory Integration and The Brain - AIT Institute 2009

Where Mind and Body Meet - Scientific American Mind 2007 - Blakeslee

You May Not Have Rhythm, but Your Brain Does - Scientific American - 2007 Nikhil Swaminathan

Rhythmic Movement - Move, Thrive, Play - 2007 - Sonia Story

There is a companion DVD available for $9.95 (plus shipping and handling) that will demonstrate how to do all the activities. I recommend purchasing it to ensure that you do the exercises that we have discussed in this book safely and correctly.

The DVD will be available on Amazon or by sending an email to cet4life@ foothill.net after December 30, 2016

nls

ABOUT THE AUTHOR

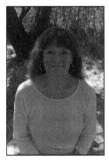 Nancy Swayzee, MES, NMT, is a seventy-seven-year-old prolific author.

Swayzee first started teaching the exercises included in her book at an aerobics studio in Colorado. After injuring her back, she focused on creating CORE exercises and sharing them with others through her book Breathworks for Your Back: Strengthening Your Back from the Inside Out. Her breathworks classes were wildly popular.

Swayzee opened a private practice of rehabilitative therapy for various injuries. She expanded her breathworks program for those with neurological disorders like Parkinson's, MS, strokes, cerebral palsy, and brain injuries. She continues to teach several classes a week.

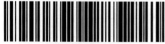

Made in the USA
San Bernardino, CA
25 January 2017